Community Psychiatry: A Reappraisal

Formulated by the
Committee on Psychiatry and Community
Group for the Advancement of Psychiatry

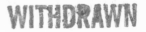

Mental Health Materials Center
30 E. 29th Street, New York, NY 10016

Library of Congress Cataloging in Publication Data
Main entry under title:

Group for the Advancement of Psychiatry. Committee on
Psychiatry and Community.

Community psychiatry.

(Publication/Group for the Advancement of Psychiatry;
v. 11, no. 113)

Includes bibliographical references.
1. Social psychiatry—Evaluation—Addresses, essays,
lectures.   2. Community mental health services—
Evaluation—Addresses, essays, lectures.   I. Group for the
Advancement of Psychiatry and Community.   II. Series:
Publication (Group for the Advancement of Psychiatry); no.
113.
[DNLM: 1. Community psychiatry.   2. Community mental
health centers—Organization and administration. WM 30.6
G882c]
RC455.C617   1983   362.2′2   83-5443
ISBN 0-910958-18-1

April, 1983, Volume XI, Publication No. 113

This is the seventh in a series of publications comprising Volume XI.

For information on availability of this publication, please contact the Mental
Health Materials Center, 30 East 29th Street, New York, NY 10016.

Manufactured in the United States of America

CONTENTS

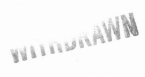

4. REAPPRAISAL AND RECOMMENDATIONS 61

STATEMENT OF PURPOSE

THE GROUP FOR THE ADVANCEMENT OF PSYCHIATRY has a
membership of approximately 300 psychiatrists, most of whom
are organized in the form of a number of working committees.
These committees direct their efforts toward the study of various
aspects of psychiatry and the application of this knowledge to the
fields of mental health and human relations.

Collaboration with specialists in other disciplines has been
and is one of GAP's working principles. Since the formation of
GAP in 1946 its members have worked closely with such other
specialists as anthropologists, biologists, economists, statisti-
cians, educators, lawyers, nurses, psychologists, sociologists,
social workers, and experts in mass communication, philosophy,
and semantics. GAP envisages a continuing program of work
according to the following aims:

1. To collect and appraise significant data in the fields of
   psychiatry, mental health, and human relations

2. To reevaluate old concepts and to develop and test new
   ones

3. To apply the knowledge thus obtained for the promotion
   of mental health and good human relations.

GAP is an independent group, and its reports represent the
composite findings and opinions of its members only, guided by
its many consultants.

COMMUNITY PSYCHIATRY: A REAPPRAISAL was formulated by the
Committee on Psychiatry and Community, which acknowledges
on page xi the participation of others in the preparation of this

v

report. The members of this committee are listed below. The following pages list the members of the other GAP committees as well as additional membership categories and current and past officers of GAP.

COMMITTEE ON PSYCHIATRY AND COMMUNITY

John J. Schwab, Louisville, Ky., Chairperson
*Lee B. Macht, Cambridge, MA
John C. Nemiah, Boston, Mass.
*Anthony F. Panzetta, Philadelphia, Pa.
*Herbert Modlin, Topeka, Kans.
Alexander S. Rogawski, Los Angeles, Calif.
John A. Talbott, New York, N.Y.
Charles B. Wilkinson, Kansas City, Mo.

COMMITTEE ON ADOLESCENCE

Warren J. Gadpaille, Englewood, Colo.,
    Chairperson
Ian A. Canino, New York, N.Y.
Harrison P. Eddy, New York, N.Y.
Sherman C. Feinstein, Highland Park, Ill.
Michael Kalogerakis, New York, N.Y.
Clarice J. Kestenbaum, New York, N.Y.
Derek Miller, Chicago, Ill.
Silvio J. Onesti, Jr., Belmont, Mass.

COMMITTEE ON AGING

Charles M. Gaitz, Houston, Tex., Chairperson
Gene D. Cohen, Rockville, Md.
Lawrence F. Greenleigh, Los Angeles, Calif.
Robert J. Nathan, Philadelphia, Pa.
George H. Pollock, Chicago, Ill.
Harvey L. Ruben, New Haven, Conn.
F. Conyers Thompson, Jr., Atlanta, Ga.

COMMITTEE ON CHILD PSYCHIATRY

John F. McDermott, Jr., Honolulu, Hawaii,
    Chairperson
Paul L. Adams, Louisville, Ky.
James M. Bell, Canaan, N.Y.

*GAP members who participated in formulation
of this report but are not longer affiliated with
this committee.

Harlow Donald Dunton, New York, N.Y.
Joseph Fischoff, Detroit, Mich.
Joseph M. Green, Madison, Wis.
John Schowalter, New Haven, Conn.
Theodore Shapiro, New York, N.Y.
Peter Tanguay, Los Angeles, Calif.
Lenore F. C. Terr, San Francisco, Calif.

COMMITTEE ON THE COLLEGE STUDENT

Kent E. Robinson, Towson, Md.,
    Chairperson
Robert L. Arnstein, Hamden, Conn.
Varda Backus, La Jolla, Calif.
Myron B. Liptzin, Chapel Hill, N.C.
Malkah Tolpin Notman, Brookline, Mass.
Gloria C. Onque, Pittsburgh, Pa.
Elizabeth Aub Reid, Cambridge, Mass.
Earle Silber, Chevy Chase, Md.

COMMITTEE ON CULTURAL PSYCHIATRY

Andrea K. Delgado, New York, N.Y.,
    Chairperson
Edward F. Foulks, Philadelphia, Pa.
Ezra E. H. Griffith, New Haven, Conn.
Pedro Ruiz, Houston, Tex.
John P. Spiegel, Waltham, Mass.
Ronald M. Wintrob, Farmington, Conn.
Joseph Yamamoto, Los Angeles, Calif.

COMMITTEE ON THE FAMILY

Henry U. Grunebaum, Cambridge, Mass.,
    Chairperson
W. Robert Beavers, Dallas, Tex.
Ellen M. Berman, Merion, Pa.
Lee Combrinck-Graham, Philadelphia, Pa.
Ira D. Glick, New York, N.Y.
Frederick Gottlieb, Los Angeles, Calif.
Charles A. Malone, Cleveland, Ohio
Joseph Satten, San Francisco, Calif.

Clarence J. Rowe, St. Paul, Minn.
John Wakefield, Saratoga, Calif.

COMMITTEE ON PSYCHOPATHOLOGY

David A. Adler, Boston, Mass., Chairperson
Wagner H. Bridger, Philadelphia, Pa.
Doyle I. Carson, Dallas, Tex.
Howard H. Goldman, San Francisco, Calif.
Douglas W. Heinrichs, Baltimore, Md.
Paul E. Huston, Iowa City, Iowa
Richard E. Renneker, Los Angeles, Calif.

COMMITTEE ON PUBLIC EDUCATION

Robert J. Campbell, New York, N.Y.,
  Chairperson
Norman L. Loux, Sellersville, Pa.
Julius Schreiber, Washington, D.C.
Miles F. Shore, Boston, Mass.
Robert A. Solow, Beverly Hills, Calif.
Kent A. Zimmerman, Berkeley, Calif.

COMMITTEE ON RESEARCH

Jerry M. Lewis, Dallas, Tex., Chairperson
John E. Adams, Gainesville, Fla.
Robert Cancro, New York, N.Y.
Stanley H. Eldred, Belmont, Mass.
John G. Gunderson, Belmont, Mass.
Morris A. Lipton, Chapel Hill, N.C.
John G. Looney, Dallas, Tex.
Charles P. O'Brien, Philadelphia, Pa.
John S. Strauss, New Haven, Conn.

COMMITTEE ON SOCIAL ISSUES

Ian A. Alger, New York, N.Y., Chairperson
Roy W. Menninger, Topeka, Kans.
William R. Beardslee, Boston, Mass.
Paul J. Fink, Philadelphia, Pa.
Henry J. Gault, Highland Park, Ill.
Roderick Gorney, Los Angeles, Calif.
Martha J. Kirkpatrick, Los Angeles, Calif.
Perry Ottenberg, Philadelphia, Pa.

COMMITTEE ON THERAPEUTIC CARE

Orlando B. Lightfoot, Boston, Mass.,
  Chairperson
Bernard Bandler, Cambridge, Mass.
Thomas E. Curtis, Chapel Hill, N.C.
Robert W. Gibson, Towson, Md.
Donald W. Hammersley, Washington, D.C.
Roberto L. Jimenez, San Antonio, Tex.
Milton Kramer, Jackson, Miss.
Melvin Sabshin, Washington, D.C.

COMMITTEE ON THERAPY

Robert Michels, New York, N.Y., Chairperson
Henry W. Brosin, Tucson, Ariz.
James S. Eaton, Jr., Rockville, Md.
Eugene B. Feigelson, Brooklyn, N.Y.
Tokoz Byram Karasu, New York, N.Y.
Andrew P. Morrison, Cambridge, Mass.
William C. Offenkrantz, Milwaukee, Wis.
Lewis L. Robbins, Glen Oaks, N.Y.
Allan D. Rosenblatt, La Jolla, Calif.

CONTRIBUTING MEMBERS

Carlos C. Alden, Jr., Buffalo, N.Y.
Charlotte G. Babcock, Pittsburgh, Pa.
Eric A. Baum, Akron, Ohio
Spencer Bayles, Houston, Tex.
Aaron T. Beck, Wynnewood, Pa.
C. Christian Beels, New York, N.Y.
Sidney Berman, Washington, D.C.
Wilfred Bloomberg, Cambridge, Mass.
Thomas L. Brannick, Imola, Calif.
H. Keith H. Brodie, Durham, N.C.
C. Martel Bryant, San Francisco, Calif.
Ewald W. Busse, Durham, N.C.
Robert N. Butler, New York, N.Y.
Eugene M. Caffey, Jr., Washington, D.C.
Paul Chodoff, Washington, D.C.
Ian L. W. Clancy, Ontario, Canada
Sanford I. Cohen, Boston, Mass.
William D. Davidson, Washington, D.C.
Lloyd C. Elam, Nashville, Tenn.
Louis C. English, Pomona, N.Y.
Raymond Feldman, Boulder, Colo.
Alfred Flarsheim, Wilmette, Ill.
Archie R. Foley, New York, N.Y.

Alan Frank, Albuquerque, N.M.
Daniel X. Freedman, Chicago, Ill.
James B. Funkhouser, Richmond, Va.
Albert J. Glass, Bethesda, Md.
Alexander Gralnick, Port Chester, N.Y.
Milton Greenblatt, Los Angeles, Calif.
John H. Greist, Indianapolis, Ind.
Roy R. Grinker, Sr., Chicago, Ill.
Lester Grinspoon, Boston, Mass.
Ernest M. Gruenberg, Baltimore, Md.
Stanley Hammons, Lexington, Ky.
Joel S. Handler, Wilmette, Ill.
Saul I. Harrison, Ann Arbor, Mich.
Peter Hartocollis, Patras, Greece
J. Cotter Hirschberg, Topeka, Kans.
Edward J. Hornick, New York, N.Y.
Joseph Hughes, Philadelphia, Pa.
Portia Bell Hume, St. Helena, Calif.
Jay Katz, New Haven, Conn.
Sheppard G. Kellam, Chicago, Ill.
Herbert L. Klemme, Stillwater, Mn.
Peter H. Knapp, Boston, Mass.
James A. Knight, New Orleans, La.
Othilda M. Krug, Cincinnati, Ohio
Robert L. Leopold, Philadelphia, Pa.
Alan I. Levenson, Tucson, Ariz.
Ruth W. Lidz, Woodbridge, Conn.
Maurice E. Linden, Philadelphia, Pa.
Reginald S. Lourie, Chevy Chase, Md.
Jeptha R. MacFarlane, Garden City, N.Y.
John A. MacLeod, Cincinnati, Ohio
Leo Madow, Philadelphia, Pa.
Sidney G. Margolin, Denver, Colo.
Peter A. Martin, Bloomfield Hills, Mich.
Ake Mattsson, New York, N.Y.
A. Louis McGarry, Great Neck, N.Y.
Alan A. McLean, New York, N.Y.
David Mendell, Houston, Tex.
Mary E. Mercer, Nyack, N.Y.
James G. Miller, Louisville, Ky.
John E. Nardini, Washington, D.C.
Joseph D. Noshpitz, Washington, D.C.
Lucy D. Ozarin, Bethesda, Md.
Bernard L. Pacella, New York, N.Y.
Norman L. Paul, Boston, Mass.
Marvin E. Perkins, Salem, Va.
Charles A. Pinderhughes, Bedford, Mass.
Seymour Pollack, Los Angeles, Calif.
David N. Ratnavale, Bethesda, Md.
Walter Reich, Rockville, Md.

Harvey L. P. Resnik, College Park, Md.
W. Donald Ross, Cincinnati, Ohio
Lester H. Rudy, Chicago, Ill.
George E. Ruff, Philadelphia, Pa.
A. John Rush, Dallas, Tex.
David S. Sanders, Los Angeles, Calif.
Donald Scherl, Brooklyn, N.Y.
Kurt O. Schlesinger, San Francisco, Calif.
Charles Shagass, Philadelphia, Pa.
Albert J. Silverman, Ann Arbor, Mich.
Justin Simon, Berkeley, Calif.
Kendon W. Smith, Valhalla, N.Y.
Benson R. Snyder, Cambridge, Mass.
David A. Soskis, Bala Cynwyd, Pa.
Jeanne Spurlock, Washington, D.C.
Alfred H. Stanton, Wellesley Hills, Mass.
Tom G. Stauffer, White Plains, N.Y.
Brandt F. Steele, Denver, Colo.
Eleanor A. Steele, Denver, Colo.
Rutherford B. Stevens, New York, N.Y.
Alan A. Stone, Cambridge, Mass.
Robert E. Switzer, Trevose, Pa.
Perry C. Talkington, Dallas, Tex.
Graham C. Taylor, Toronto, Canada
Bryce Templeton, Philadelphia, Pa.
Prescott W. Thompson, Beaverton, Oreg.
Harvey J. Tompkins, New York, N.Y.
Lucia E. Tower, Chicago, Ill.
Joseph P. Tupin, Sacramento, Calif.
John A. Turner, San Francisco, Calif.
Montague Ullman, Ardsley, N.Y.
Gene L. Usdin, New Orleans, La.
Warren T. Vaughan, Jr., Portola Valley, Calif.
Robert S. Wallerstein, San Francisco, Calif.
Andrew S. Watson, Ann Arbor, Mich.
Bryant M. Wedge, Washington, D.C.
Joseph B. Wheelwright, Kentfield, Calif.
Robert L. Williams, Houston, Tex.
Paul Tyler Wilson, Bethesda, Md.
Sherwyn M. Woods, Los Angeles, Calif.
Stanley F. Yolles, Stony Brook, N.Y.
Israel Zwerling, Philadelphia, Pa.

LIFE MEMBERS

C. Knight Aldrich, Charlottesville, Va.
Bernard Bandler, Cambridge, Mass.
Walter E. Barton, Hartland, Vt.
Ivan C. Berlien, Coral Gables, Fla.
Murray Bowen, Chevy Chase, Md.

COMMITTEE ACKNOWLEDGMENTS

We are exceedingly fortunate to have had three of the leaders in the field of community mental health as consultants to our Committee. Leona S. Bachrach, Ph.D., was our regular Blanche F. Ittleson Consultant; she worked with the Committee during the entire time required to prepare the report. H. Warren Dunham, Ph.D., a pioneer in psychiatric sociology and in community psychiatry, gave us a review of 50 years of activities in the Community Mental Health movement that stimulated our thinking. Jack Zusman, M.D., formerly a faculty member in the Program for Training Community Psychiatrists at Columbia University (1962–1966) and Director of the Center for Epidemiologic Studies in Washington in the 1960s, supplied us with valuable information about the development of the Federally-funded Community Mental Health Center program.

Three Ginsburg Fellows worked with the Committee on the report. They are John I. Walker, M.D., Richard Whitten-Stovall, M.D., and Rebecca Potter, M.D.—a Fellow during this academic year. Dr. Whitten-Stovall returned to our meetings as a Post-Fellow Guest.

John J. Schwab, *Chairperson*
Committee on Psychiatry and Community

1

INTRODUCTION

In 1964, community psychiatry was proclaimed the third psychiatric revolution, equal in significance to Pinel's unchaining of the insane and Freud's discovery of psychoanalysis. It was described optimistically in the 1967 GAP Report, EDUCATION FOR COMMUNITY PSYCHIATRY, as

> ". . . an evolving aspect of psychiatry in which the psychiatrist accepts responsibility within a population . . . for promotion of mental health, prevention, early case finding, and treatment, . . . an emerging subspecialty of psychiatry."[1]

But not everyone shared the enthusiasm for community psychiatry. Kubie feared that community psychiatry would "suffer the fate of all good intentions not guided by mature judgment and experience" and that psychiatrists might be misled by its illusions and practices.[2] In calling it "The Newest Therapeutic Bandwagon," Warren Dunham expressed skepticism about its future.[3] He viewed it as mainly a reorganization of mental health services geared toward work with patients, their families, and supportive agencies in the community. Dunham doubted the "adequacy of our knowledge to develop significant techniques for treating social collectives or for developing techniques on the community level that will really result in a reduction of mental disturbances in the community."[4]

The skeptics were closer to the truth in their predictions than the enthusiasts. During the 1970s, community psychiatry not only failed to emerge as a subspecialty, but its status became progressively more controversial. By the beginning of the 1980s, optimism about the Federal Community Mental Health Centers had turned to despair. Their very existence was in jeopardy and psychiatry's role in them had become clouded and tenuous.

To add to the difficulties, distinctions among (a) "community psychiatry," (b) "the Community Mental Health movement," and (c) the "Community Mental Health Center (CMHC) program" have been blurred. Even Kubie did not distinguish among them and, at least by implication, submerged the concept of community psychiatry into that of community mental health. Many authorities did not recognize that community psychiatry had a long history of achievement even before the advent of the Community Mental Health movement.

(a) *Community psychiatry* is the application of the theory and practice of psychiatry in noninstitutional and relatively nontraditional settings. It has the following characteristics:

- It is based on the assumption that sociocultural conditions significantly influence the definition, manifestations, and course of mental illness.
- It studies the role of the social environment in mental illness.
- It is concerned with the organization and delivery of mental health services.
- It uses social and environmental measures to prevent mental illness and to treat and care for those who develop mental disorders.
- It supplies treatment and care as close as possible to the patient's residence or workplace.
- It utilizes community resources to extend services beyond the more conventional psychiatric treatment programs.

(b) We view the *Community Mental Health movement* as a historical development spearheaded by professionals from a number of disciplines, by concerned public figures, and by citizen advocates who have taken sociopolitical action to:

- Provide care for the mentally ill close to their homes, and
- Direct efforts and funds toward the prevention of mental illness by implementing the principles of "mental hygiene" and by improving the quality of life in the community.

(c) The *CMHC program* refers to the Federally-funded CMHCs developed under the auspices of Federal legislation. As a new approach to mental health care, it created Centers to provide mandated services to the mentally ill in the community and to prevent mental illness according to guidelines and regulations formulated mainly by Federal agencies.

Concern about the state and the fate of the CMHC program stems both from anxiety about the quality of care for the seriously mentally ill in the community and from perplexity about psychiatry's role in the program. These concerns are compounded by uncertainty about the fiscal future of the program and its tenuous, if not erratic, relationship to medical and social resources.

The often disastrous consequences of deinstitutionalization have heightened apprehension about the effectiveness of CMHCs.* Many mentally-ill persons are merely lodged in nursing or in board-and-care homes in the community where they receive little or no mental health care. Others are being crowded into penal institutions[6] or are roaming at large where they become victims or victimizers. For the most part CMHCs are not taking adequate care of the seriously and chronically mentally-ill patients.[7]

Psychiatry's concurrent decline of interest in the CMHC program is demonstrated by the diminishing emphasis on com-

---

*In accord with Bachrach's definition, deinstitutionalization is the eschewal of traditional institutional settings (particularly State mental hospitals) and the concurrent expansion of community-based facilities for the care of chronic mental patients.[5]

munity psychiatry in residency training programs and the decreasing number of psychiatrists working in CMHCs. Between 1970 and 1976, the average number of psychiatrists working in CMHCs fell from 6.8 to 4.3; in contrast, the number of social workers rose from 9.1 to 13.0.[8]

To obtain a clearer understanding of the nature and status of community psychiatry in the 1980s, in Chapter 2 we shall look at its history and at the evolution of the Community Mental Health movement. In Chapter 3 we shall examine the basic assumptions held by proponents of the Community Mental Health movement that influenced the development of the CMHC program, guided its implementation and operations, and thus affected its current status. In Chapter 4 we shall assess the failures and successes of the CMHC program and present our conclusions and recommendations. We hope that this scrutiny will clarify community psychiatry's often ambiguous position and will support our recommendations for better care of patients and for better training of psychiatrists and other mental health personnel.

REFERENCES

1. Group for the Advancement of Psychiatry. Committee on Medical Education. *Education for Community Psychiatry*. Report No. 64. New York: Mental Health Materials Center, Inc., 1967, p. 494.
2. Kubie, L. Pitfalls of community psychiatry, *Archives of General Psychiatry,* 18(3):257–266, 1968.
3. Dunham, W. Community psychiatry: The newest therapeutic bandwagon. In *Social Psychiatry*, A. Kiev (Ed.). Vol. 1. New York: Science House, Inc., 1966, pp. 217–239.
4. Ibid., p. 237.
5. Bachrach, L. L. *Deinstitutionalization: An Analytical Review and Sociological Perspective*. Rockville, MD: NIMH, 1976.

6. Bonowitz, J. C., and E. B. Guy. Commitment procedures on prison psychiatric services, *American Journal of Psychiatry*, 136(8): 1045–1048, 1979.
7. Sharfstein, S. S. Will community mental health survive in the 1980s? *American Journal of Psychiatry*, 135(11): 1363–1367, 1978.
8. *Provisional Data on Federally Funded Community Mental Health Centers, 1976–1977.* Rockville, MD: NIMH Division of Biometry and Epidemiology, Survey and Reports Branch, May, 1978.

2

THE HISTORICAL BACKGROUND

Whether mental patients receive better treatment in a hospital or in a community setting is a question that is centuries old. Cultural, political, economic, and individual biases—rather than studies of their relative merits—have influenced advocacy of one or the other treatment setting. A brief survey of the history of the care of mental patients, of the evolution of the Community Mental Health movement, and of the development of the CMHC program is necessary to assess some of these factors and to appraise the status of community psychiatry.

EARLY HISTORY

In Western society during the Middle Ages, the mentally ill were tolerated in the community as long as they were quiet and harmless. Considered odd, but not ostracized, they were cared for by their families or by religious institutions. In the sixteenth and seventeenth centuries, concurrent with the disappearance of feudalism and the emergence of nationalism, public attitudes toward the mentally ill changed. In this era of the Great Confinement, the mentally ill along with many other unfortunates— cripples, indigents, and those on the fringes of society—were seen as a threat to the social fabric and were institutionalized, ostensibly to protect the community from their baneful influence.

During the eighteenth century, the proliferation of unregulated madhouses aroused public indignation. Many were merely prison-like institutions operated by individuals who sought to profit from the infirmities of their charges. Too often, inmates were subjected to indignities and cruelties. But here and there, an enlightened Pinel or Tuke demonstrated that a humane and caring environment could restore severely afflicted and chronic mental patients to reason and to normal living.

1855, Edward Jarvis, Chairman of the Commission on Lunacy for the State of Massachusetts, wrote about conditions in that state.

> Men of disordered mind, when they need a change of air or scene, cannot go to a hotel, or boarding house, or even a friend's private house, as those can who are merely invalids in body. They require more caution, forbearance and oversight, and many of them are annoying to those who are about them. They must, therefore, go to houses, places, or people devoted to their care and prepared to give them the needful attention and watchfulness.[1]

He argued that properly-run institutions were helpful to patients and that it was economically advantageous for the state to increase the number of hospital beds for mental patients. This assumption had inspired earlier nineteenth century reformers, notably Dorothea Dix, to recommend construction of a number of new, publicly-supported hospitals.[2] A serendipitous benefit was that these government–funded asylums attracted a cadre of staff physicians who soon acquired special knowledge of the nature and treatment of mental disorders.

During this period, both physicians and the public believed that the asylum was the best place to treat the mentally ill. Well before the beginning of the twentieth century, however, asylums were no longer treating patients actively. They were serving mainly as depositories for the swelling numbers of the chronic mentally ill. Notwithstanding frequent exposés and campaigns for reform, asylums continued to exist primarily as places where the mentally disordered could be kept out of sight.

THE DEVELOPMENT OF COMMUNITY PSYCHIATRY

Prior to 1900, two sets of developments stimulated interest in community psychiatry. One was the philosophical shift from Social Darwinism to Progressivism that abetted much of the social reform at the turn of the century. Social Darwinism suggested that mental illness was a biological failure of adaptation; isolation of its victims in asylums would prevent propagation or "contagion."[3] In contrast, Progressivism suggested environmental explanations; mental illness resulted from a "bad" childhood, slum conditions, poor family background, and the "incorrect" attitudes of others.[4]

The other development was the beginning use of alternatives to the asylum. During the nineteenth century, American psychiatry became interested in such experiments as J. M. Galt's Farm of St. Anne and the 1885 Massachusetts program for boarding mental patients in private homes.[5,6] In the 1890s, Peterson and Chapin espoused a new type of facility—the psychopathic hospital located in the community and dedicated to active treatment that would involve family, friends, and local medical practitioners.[7,8] The concept of aftercare also began to receive attention; its implementation required the efforts of persons functioning as social workers who collaborated with psychiatrists.[9]

In the first decade of this century, three influences moved American psychiatry closer to the community and laid the foundation for the Community Mental Health movement. Foremost was the Mental Hygiene movement initiated by Clifford Beer's publication of *A Mind That Found Itself*[10] which exposed the wretched conditions in mental hospitals. In 1909, Beers organized the National Committee for Mental Hygiene to collect data on mental health programs to educate the public, and to advocate programs and legislation for improving mental institutions. In addition to its efforts to arouse public concern about mental illness, the Committee's most significant contribution to the

Community Mental Health movement was its insistence on involving nonmedical personnel in patient care and on using interdisciplinary groups to establish demonstration clinics and promote interdisciplinary training.

The second influence was the Public Health program advocated by Adolf Meyer[11] which delineated many of the tenets and components of community psychiatry: the important role of the social environment in the development and course of mental illness; an integrated program of prevention, treatment and aftercare; participation by family physicians; the organization of care within defined geographic districts; and education of the public about mental illness.

The third influence was the Child Guidance movement. In 1909, William Healy, encouraged by the new psychoanalytic concepts, established the Chicago Juvenile Psychopathic Institute to make recommendations to referring agencies for indirect services as well as for direct treatment of children. Healy reported that adult psychopathology and criminality could be prevented by early attention to children at risk.[12] Inspired by his work, the Commonwealth Fund provided a grant in 1920 to establish Child Guidance Clinics designed to acquaint parents and teachers with proper child-rearing techniques and thus prevent psychiatric morbidity and delinquency in adults.

Meanwhile, the miserable conditions in the public mental hospitals spurred the search for alternatives to asylums. Pioneer community psychiatry programs included such innovations as: tent treatment on Ward's Island (1901), the probationary discharge of chronic patients into the community under the supervision of social services (1904), the cottage system (1905), the travelling clinic in New York State (1909), and the first outpatient clinics (1912).

More of the fundamental components of community psychiatry appeared in the early decades of this century. Massachusetts was divided into twenty districts to enable "each hospital to reach out in the community and be responsible for the mental health of the district covered by each." [13] Following his visits to World War I battlefield facilities, Thomas Salmon recommended short-term crisis intervention based on the concepts of immediacy (no waiting lists), proximity (clinics located near patients' homes), and expectancy (anticipation of recovery). [14] By the time the war ended, heightened public awareness of the magnitude of the number of mentally ill stimulated further developments in community psychiatry and the evolution of the more widespread Community Mental Health movement. Psychiatric social work attained status as a profession shortly before the end of World War I. In 1922, the American Sociological Association initiated linkages between psychiatry and the social sciences by establishing a psychiatric section entitled, "Psychic Factors in Social Conditions." [15]

A change in social philosophies during the 1920s and 1930s—away from Emerson's self-reliance toward concerns about social structure and function—provided a rationale for community rather than personal solutions to mental illness and other social problems. For example, in "The Society as the Patient," [16] L. K. Frank attributed crime, prostitution, mental disorders, and other ills to social injustices, not to disturbances in the individual. Some theorists and activists advocated social engineering—manipulating the "social, economic, and political environment," [17] in the interests of mental health.

The proliferation of Federal assistance programs during the Great Depression reflected these radically changed attitudes; the public began to believe that the Government should be responsible for all of the disadvantaged. [18] In 1930, the United States Public Health Service expanded the Narcotic Division into the Division of Mental Hygiene which, in 1949, became the National Institute of Mental Health.

Efforts to move away from asylum psychiatry continued during the 1920s and 1930s. The first psychiatric units were opened in general hospitals and about 400 "mental clinics" were established "to involve families and communities in prevention (of mental illness) and the care of the mentally ill." [19] Developments abroad during the 1930s probably had even more impact on community psychiatry and on the evolution of the Community Mental Health movement than did those in the United States. Great Britain enacted the Mental Health Treatment Act that allowed voluntary hospitalization. The open ward policy was re-established in England for the first time since the beginning of the Era of Moral Treatment more than a century earlier. At Marlborough Day Hospital, Bierer established the Therapeutic Social Club for the seriously and chronically mentally ill. [20] The first day hospital was opened in Moscow. And Querido inaugurated the travelling home care program in Amsterdam. [21]

World War II spurred additional moves toward community services. The public was both surprised and alarmed by the prevalence of mental illness in the military services. On pre-induction screenings, 1,875,000 men were found to be emotionally unfit for service and 850,000 (40% of *all* dischargees) were released from active service because of mental illness. [22-24] The Government responded dramatically. The Mental Health Act of 1946 created the National Institute of Mental Health in order to have "the traditional public health approach applied to the mental health field" [25] and the Veterans' Administration established special mental health services.

Even before such Federal initiatives took effect, developments in American psychiatry shortly after World War II began to change the mental health system. Some of the most prominent were the increased private office practice of psychiatry, Erich Lindemann's development of crisis theory and intervention, the opening of the first day hospital in North America at the Allen Memorial Institute in Montreal, and the establishment of an expatient social rehabilitation program—Fountain House—in New York City. [26-28] Other notable moves toward community psychiatry were: the breaking up of large State hospitals in Kansas and New York into decentralized and, later, geographically-related units; the establishment of satellite hospitals in the community in Connecticut and Massachusetts; and the integration of County and State services to provide precare, inpatient care, and aftercare in Dutchess County, New York.[29]

Again, developments *abroad* stimulated the growth of community services in the late 1940s and early 1950s. In Great Britain, the open ward policy was just one part of a broader program aimed at decreasing symptoms by treating patients as responsible persons. Maxwell Jones popularized the therapeutic community.[30] The British National Health Act of 1948 ensured that relatives could obtain a patient's discharge unless the patient was considered to be dangerous. In Israel, Gerald Caplan established a community consultation program for social workers aimed at the prevention of mental illness in children through intervention with their mothers.[31] In France, Paul Sivadon advocated sociotherapy, resocialization, and a unit system for hospitals.[32]

Thus, various community psychiatry concepts and programs were coalescing and soon became articulated plans. As early as 1952, a plan drafted by a blue-ribbon WHO committee spelled out the functions of the community mental hospital—outpatient treatment, part-time treatment, rehabilitation, research, and community education.[33] But the fervor of the 1960s to serve the disadvantaged in our nation would be required to transform the plans into action.

In the meantime, leaders of the American Psychiatric Association and The Group for the Advancement of Psychiatry, such as Appel, Solomon, and William Menninger, issued calls for the implementation of community psychiatry programs.[34, 35] Congress responded in 1955 by establishing the Joint Commission on Mental Illness and Health which was charged to make recommendations for a comprehensive program for the care of the mentally ill.

A rapid series of developments in psychiatry during the 1950s accelerated the move toward the community. Some of these were: Caplan's theory of community consultation, halfway houses and night and weekend hospitals, travelling clinics, vocational rehabilitation for mental patients, 24-hour emergency walk-in services and suicide prevention centers, community clinics for State hospital patients, the use of community agencies (e.g., schools and churches) as mental health extenders, and the search for alternatives to hospitalization.[36-43]

The belief that mental illness reflected environmental influences led to interventions in schools and playgrounds. The longstanding shortage of mental health professionals was compensated for, in part, by the burgeoning use of paraprofessionals and indigenous workers. Starting in 1955, coincident with the early use of chlorpromazine and concomitant developments in community psychiatry, the patient census in New York State mental hospitals dropped for the first time in a century.

Research in social and community psychiatry flourished. In 1954, Stanton and Schwartz[44] described the effects of staff dissension on patient behavior. In 1958, Hollingshead and Redlich[45] showed that disparate treatments were provided to different socioeconomic groups. In the same year, Caudill[46] stressed the importance of group dynamics in the hospital ward. In 1959, Leighton and his coworkers presented findings showing that community disorganization was associated with mental illness.[47] In 1961, Goffman[48] painted a devastating picture of life in mental hospitals. In 1962, Srole and his colleagues[49] reported that only 18 percent of the Midtown residents were both symptom-free and functionally unimpaired. Thus, extensive research activity increased the momentum toward community-based services. Musto states that research findings documented the link between the environment and health, demonstrated the immense need for more mental health workers, and offered a "gigantic opportunity for social progress."[50]

The 1960s were heady times for social reform as evidenced by programs for neighborhood health centers and model cities. Heightened concern for the disadvantaged and oppressed led to the War on Poverty, the Civil Rights Movement, and various liberation fronts. The Federal Government attempted to achieve "maximum feasible participation" on the part of the citizenry.[51] Optimism reigned and a spirit of hope swept mental health circles. Many believed that a Federally-budgeted program could be designed to deal with almost any social or economic problem— an attitude later characterized by former Budget Director Schultz as the "throwing money at problems attitude."[52]

The Levines[53] have pointed out that, historically, psychiatry swings between sociopolitical conservatism—when problems are deemed intrapsychic and treatment is geared to the individual—and sociopolitical liberalism—when problems are thought to be environmental and social intervention is aimed toward reducing the incidence of disease. During conservative times, resources are used mainly to provide treatment to the manifestly mentally ill. But during liberal eras, the prevailing beliefs are that primary prevention is attainable, that group action can solve problems, and that the human resources are greater than just the number of professionals in the mental health disciplines. Zusman noted that the philosophy of community psychiatry paralleled Kennedy's "Camelot"—"Optimistic, romantic and liberal . . . social conditions cause mental illness so [one must] change social conditions."[54]

In 1961, the final report of the Joint Commission, *Action for Mental Health*,[55] called for: more money for mental hospitals and research; the establishment of community clinics connected with general hospitals that would serve no more than 50,000 persons; expanded community services; the location of psychiatric services near patients' homes; community education to foster prevention; and greatly increased numbers of non-professional mental health workers. Although a few critics, such as Caplan,[56] complained that the Report favored services to ill adults over prevention, most authorities believed that the recommendations were balanced.

President Kennedy's 1963 Congressional Message on Mental Health, however, presented a "bold new approach," a drastic change in emphasis—away from the hospital-based services recommended by the Joint Commission and toward the development of "comprehensive community mental health centers." [57] His message was followed by the passage of legislation, PL88-164 in 1963 [58] and PL89-105 in 1965 [59] (the CMHC Act and Amendment), that established the CMHC program. The Joint Commission had recommended improved State hospital care, early intervention, provision for aftercare, travelling clinics, and psychiatry in the community. [60] However, in its bureaucratic journey from Report to Congressional legislation, the travelling clinic became a "center" serving a "community." Although community psychiatry had developed major concepts and approaches, it was soon overshadowed by the Community Mental Health movement which took tangible form with the launching of the CMHC program. By failing to mandate aftercare as a required service, the legislation allowed CMHCs to concentrate on the less severely disturbed. In 1967, Freedman presciently wrote,

> There is a danger that in paying increased attention to the socially deviant and the neurotic in the community the traditional responsibility of psychiatry for caring for the severely disturbed or psychotic will be minimized or abandoned. [61]

MENTAL HEALTH OR ILLNESS?

Definitions of mental health fall into several broad categories— the absolute and the relative. An example of the former is the World Health Organization's statement that health "is a state of complete physical, mental, and social well-being, and not merely the absence of disease and infirmity." [62] In contrast, the relativistic point of view is expressed by Laughlin who views mental health and illness as conditions on a continuum: "the 'normal' imperceptibly merges into the borderline, and the borderline into the

neurotic."[63] Still another is the traditional definition of health as
the absence of disease.

In the 1950s, when the Community Mental Health movement
was taking shape, definitions of mental health tended to emphasize both emotional and social well-being, and, at least implicitly,
well-being was equated with adaptation and social adjustment.
Karl Menninger's 1953 statement epitomized a long-standing
view of mental health:

> Let us define mental health as the adjustment of human beings to each
> other and to the world about them with a maximum of effectiveness and
> happiness.[64]

Such an idealistic definition of mental health—embodying
adaptation, social adjustment, and even happiness—established
a goal that had a broad popular appeal. The yearning for such an
ideal condition gave impetus to the poorly conceptualized,
hastily designed, untested, pell-mell rush into CMHC programs.

The emphasis on mental health also led to such concepts as
Thomas Szasz's "myth of mental illness." In 1960, he declared
that, far from being an entity, mental illness was merely a
deviation from the norm established by "psychosocial, ethical,
and legal concepts."[65] Other writers also decried the effects of
labeling and social control processes on the cause and treatment
of mental disorders. Parsons maintained:

> We are more likely to interpret a difficulty in an individual's fulfilling
> social role expectations as a disturbance in capacity, i.e., an illness, than
> is true in other types of societies with other types of value systems.[66]

The emphasis on mental health, the equating of mental health
with adaptation and social adjustment, and the view that mental
illness is a social phenomenon have had far-reaching consequences. One of the most significant and problematic was that a
higher priority was given to the prevention of mental illness than
to the treatment of the mentally disturbed.

THE CMHC PROGRAM

The legislation creating CMHCs combined many elements of community psychiatry programs developed during the preceding 100 years:

- CMHCs were intended to provide comprehensive care and continuity of care.
- Services would be accessible and available to persons of all ages and diagnostic categories.
- The centers would be accountable to the community.
- Information would be exchanged among agencies.
- Patients would be transferred within the system.

The originally mandated five essential services were: inpatient, outpatient, partial hospitalization, 24-hour emergency care, and community consultation and education. Five desirable but optional services were: specialized diagnostic services, precare and aftercare, rehabilitation, training, and research and evaluation.

In the early 1960s it was envisioned that about 1500 CMHCs throughout the nation—a new mental health care system—would not only solve the problem of mental illness and eliminate State hospitals, but also, promote mental health and well-being. Although the CMHC program was conceptualized as one that would decentralize responsibility, in reality, care for the mentally ill was funded initially and regulated subsequently by the Federal Government. Paradoxically, the attempt to move responsibility for the mentally ill from the national to the local level occurred at a time when the taxing power of the Federal Government increased greatly while that of most local governments decreased. Also, further development of the CMHC program, as well as other social and community programs, was hampered by our nation's complex financial and social difficulties during the Vietnam era.

The CMHCs developed gradually, following to some extent a complicated priority formula designed to provide services soonest to areas in greatest need. Although many centers appeared to be accomplishing some of their treatment goals, at the same time they were running into problems. Some problems were that:

- The centers tended to reinforce the dual system of mental health care—one for private and another for public patients—because of budget limitations, the shortage of trained personnel, and the view that treatment of the disadvantaged often required disadvantaged personnel.
- The centers relied increasingly on the use of inadequately trained and relatively inexperienced counsellors and therapists.
- The centers paid insufficient attention to the needs of the severely mentally ill and sometimes neglected, or provided substandard services for, chronic patients.
- The centers' attempts to take care of the chronically ill were compounded by precipitate and indiscriminate deinstitutionalization, often in the absence of community resources for alternative types of care; and
- Public opposition to center activities was supported by fears that the presence of the mentally ill and of facilities for care in the community would exert deleterious influences on others, lower property values, and limit the coping abilities of communities.

In the 1970s, the difficulties of the CMHC program grew. Only about one-half of the intended numbers of the centers had opened and it was becoming evident that they were failing to provide adequate care for the severely and chronically mentally ill and to prevent mental illness. Also, many CMHCs were unable to coordinate often scarce community resources or to develop needed back-up for and by the State hospital system. The lack of community financial support to replace Federal funding and unexpectedly great competition for public funds from private and other public agencies led to programmatic changes toward revenue producing services and a shrinkage of services for the destitute. The centers began to lose their medical identity and many disillusioned psychiatrists left the centers to engage in private practice.

In short, when faced with the realities of the mental illness problem and political and economic exigencies, the Community Mental Health movement—in operation as the CMHC program—found that it could neither promote mental health nor provide adequate treatment for the mentally ill, and that it could not deal with communities as had been hoped. In 1977, a new Commission on Mental Health was established by President Carter, in part to rectify some of the major problems encountered by CMHCs. Its 1978 Report documented the difficulties we have listed and led to the passage of the Community Mental Health Systems Act of 1980[67] which made the states responsible for coordinating and regulating CMHCs and other mental health services. It broadened eligibility for Federal funds (which were to have been channeled through the States), suggested solutions to the problems of the chronically ill, and recommended that the mental health system be viewed as encompassing a wider range of facilities and services than just the CMHCs.

Whether the changes advocated by the Mental Health Systems Act will materialize is doubtful. As of early 1983, the Act had not been funded and it was widely rumored that the Reagan Administration might seek to repeal it. No alternative programs had been suggested and the only certainty was that the level of Federal funding for mental health programs would be drastically reduced and probably channeled to the states as limited block grants for human services including CMHCs.

REFERENCES

1. Jarvis, E. *Report on Insanity and Idiocy in Massachusetts by the Commission on Lunacy.* Boston: Wm. White, Printer to the State, 1855, p. 106.
2. Grob, G. N. *Mental Institutions in America: Social Policy to 1875.* New York: The Free Press, 1973.
3. Rossi, A. Some pre-World War II antecedents of community mental health theory and practice, *Mental Hygiene*, 46:78–98, 1962.
4. Musto, D. The Community Mental Health Movement in historical perspective. In *An Assessment of the Community Mental Health Movement*, W. E. Barton and C. J. Sanborn (Eds.). Lexington, MA: Lexington Books, 1975, p. 2.
5. Galt, J. M. The farm of St. Anne, *American Journal of Insanity*, 11:352–357, 1855.
6. Copp, O. Further experience in family care of the insane in Massachusetts, *American Journal of Insanity*, 63:361–365, 1907.
7. See citation 3.
8. *The Institutional Care of the Insane in the United States and Canada*, Vol. 1, H. M. Hurd (Ed.). Baltimore: Johns Hopkins Press, 1946, pp. 258–280.
9. A century of debate surrounding community care, *Hospital & Community Psychiatry*, 27:490, 1976.
10. Beers, C. *A Mind That Found Itself.* New York: Doubleday, 1908.
11. Meyer, A. Organizing the community for the protection of its mental life, *Survey*, 34:557–560, 1915.
12. Healy, W. *The Individual Delinquent.* Boston: Little Brown, 1915.
13. Grob, G. N. *The State and the Mentally Ill: A History of Worcester State Hospital in Massachusetts, 1830–1920.* Chapel Hill, NC: University of North Carolina Press, 1966, p. 350.
14. Salmon, T. W., and N. Fenton. The American expeditionary forces. In *The Medical Department of the United States Army in the World War, Neuropsychiatry.* Vol. 10. Washington, DC: USGPO, 1929.
15. See citation 3.
16. Frank, L. K. The society as the patient, *American Journal of Sociology*, 42:335–344, 1936.
17. Caplan, G., and R. B. Caplan. Development of community psychiatry concepts. In *Comprehensive Textbook of Psychiatry*, A. M.

Freedman and H. I. Kaplan (Eds.). Baltimore: Williams and Wilkins Co., 1967, pp. 1499–1516.

18. See citation 4, p. 7.
19. Jarrett, M. C. Mental clinics. In *Clinics, Hospital and Health Centers*, M. M. Davis (Ed.). New York: Harper, 1927, pp. 426–452.
20. Bierer, J. The Marlborough experiment. In *Handbook of Community Psychiatry and Community Mental Health*, L. Bellak (Ed.). New York: Grune and Stratton, 1964, pp. 223–228.
21. Querido, A. Early diagnosis and treatment services. In *Milbank Memorial Fund: The Elements of a Community Mental Health Program*. New York: Milbank Memorial Fund, 1956, pp. 158–181.
22. Felix, R. H. Mental illness: Psychiatry in prospect, *American Journal of Psychiatry*, 103:600–604, 1947.
23. Whittington, H. B. *Psychiatry in the American Community*. New York: International Universities Press, 1966, p. 15.
24. Mora, G. Recent American psychiatric developments (since 1939). In *Handbook of American Psychiatry*, S. Arieti (Ed.). New York: Basic Books, Inc., 1959, pp. 40–41.
25. Glasscote, R., D. Sanders, H. M. Forstenzer, and A. Foley. *The Community Mental Health Center: An Analysis of Existing Models*. Washington, D. C.: Joint Information Service, 1964.
26. Lindemann, E. Symptomatology and management of acute grief, *American Journal of Psychiatry*, 101:141–148, 1944.
27. See citation 3.
28. Becker, A., M. Murphy, and M. Greenblatt. Recent advances in community psychiatry, *New England Journal of Medicine*, 272:621–626, 1965.
29. Ibid.
30. Jones, M. *The Therapeutic Community*. New York: Basic Books, Inc., 1953.
31. Caplan, G. A community approach to preventive psychiatry—a conceptual framework. In *An Approach to Community Mental Health*. New York: Grune and Stratton, 1961, pp. 1–31.
32. Sivadon, P. Techniques of sociotherapy. In *Symposium on Preventive and Social Psychiatry*. Washington, DC: Walter Reed Army Institute of Research, 1957, pp. 457–464.
33. See citation 22.
34. Appel, K. The present challenge of psychiatry, *American Journal of Psychiatry*, 111:1012, 1954.

35. Solomon, H. The American Psychiatric Association in relation to American psychiatry, *American Journal of Psychiatry*, 115:1–9, 1958.

36. Caplan, G. *Principles of Preventive Psychiatry*. New York: Basic Books, Inc., 1964.

37. See citation 28.

38. See citation 20.

39. Brown, W. H., L. H. Takraff, B. H. Gostes, and C. N. Madsen. Using community agencies in the treatment program of a traveling child guidance clinic, *Mental Hygiene*, 41:372–377, 1957.

40. Bellak, L. The comprehensive community psychiatry program at City Hospital. See citation 20.

41. Sampson, H., D. Ross, B. Engle, and E. Livson. Feasibility of community clinic treatment for State mental hospitals, AMA *Archives of Neurological Psychiatry*, 80:71–77, 1958.

42. *Action for Mental Health. The Final Report on the Joint Commission on Mental Illness and Health*. New York: Basic Books, Inc., 1961.

43. Hunt, R. C. Community responsibility for mental health in Britain, The Netherlands, and New York State, *Psychiatric Quarterly,* 30:684–697, 1956.

44. Stanton, A. H., and M. S. Schwartz. *The Mental Hospital*. New York: Basic Books, Inc., 1954.

45. Hollingshead, A. B., and F. C. Redlich. *Social Class and Mental Illness: A Community Study*. New York: John Wiley and Sons, 1958.

46. Caudill, W. Problems of leadership in the overt and covert social structure of psychiatric hospitals. See citation 32, pp. 345–364.

47. Leighton, A. H. *My Name is Legion*. New York: Basic Books, Inc., 1959.

48. Goffman, E. *Asylums*. New York: Doubleday and Co., 1961.

49. Srole, L., T. S. Langner, S. T. Michael, et al. *Mental Health in the Metropolis. The Midtowm Manhattan Study*. Vol. 1 in the Thomas A. C. Rennie Series in Social Psychiatry. New York: McGraw-Hill, 1962.

50. See citation 4, p. 9.

51. Rubin, L. B. Maximum feasible participation: The origins, implications and current Status, *American Academy of Political and Social Sciences,* 385:14–29, 1969.

52. Schultz, C. L. The public use of private interest, *Harpers*, May 1977, pp. 43–62.

53. Levine, M., and A. Levine. *A Social History of the Helping Services.* New York: Appleton-Century-Crofts, 1970.
54. Zusman, J. The philosophic basis for a community and social psychiatry. See citation 4, pp. 27–28.
55. See citation 42.
56. See citation 36.
57. Kennedy, J. F. Message from the President of the United States relative to mental illness and mental retardation, *American Journal of Psychiatry,* 120:729–737, 1964.
58. *Public Law 88-164. The Mental Retardation Facilities and Community Mental Health Centers Construction Act of 1963.* Washington, DC: USGPO, 1963.
59. *Public Law 89-105. The Mental Retardation Facilities and Community Mental Health Centers Construction Act Amendments of 1965.* Washington, DC: USGPO, 1965.
60. Ewalt, J. R. Recommendations for a national mental health program: Summary. See citation 42, pp. vii–xxxiii.
61. Freedman, A. M. Historical and political roots of the Community mental Health Centers Act, *American Journal of Orthopsychiatry,* 37:487–494, April, 1967.
62. World Health Organization. *The First Ten Years of the World Health Organization.* Geneva: WHO, 1958, p. 459.
63. Laughlin, H. L. *The Neuroses.* Washington, DC: Butterworths, 1967, p. 2.
64. Menninger, K. A. Quoted in Anderson, C. L., R. F. Morton, and L. W. Green. *Community Health.* St. Louis: The C. V. Mosby Co., 1978, p. 93.
65. Szasz, T. The myth of mental illness, *American Psychology,* 15:113–118, 1960.
66. Parsons, T. *Social Structure and Personality.* New York: The Free Press of Glencoe, 1964, p. 291.
67. McDonald, M. C. President signs MH Systems Act into law, *Psychiatric News,* XB(21):1, 1980.

3

ASSUMPTIONS—
IMPLEMENTATION AND OUTCOME

Both explicitly and implicitly, the CMHC program was based on nine major assumptions: (1) care in the community is less expensive than care in the hospital; (2) care in the community is better than care in the hospital; (3) comprehensive care is a desirable and necessary goal that can be achieved in the community; (4) continuity of care is beneficial; (5) the designation of catchment areas enhances the provision of services; (6) accessibility to mental health services is essential; (7) the social environment produces mental illness; (8) preventive efforts reduce the incidence and prevalence of mental illness; and (9) local responsibility and control is necessary to ensure the success of CMHCs. Many of these assumptions were considered to have *prima facie* validity, but they had been neither examined carefully nor tested scientifically. We shall describe their rationale and implementation, examine their validity, and evaluate their significance for community psychiatry in the future.

Care in the Community is Less Expensive Than Care in the Hospital

It was widely believed that closing mental hospitals and providing care in community facilities would reduce the "cost of mental illness." But there have been few data available either to support or to refute this belief. Although mental hospitals were expensive to build and staff, economic as well as humanitarian considerations led to the widespread construction of a large number of them in the middle of the nineteenth century. In his famous

1855 *Report*, Jarvis emphasized that hospital treatment was both effective and economically sound.

> Insanity, if not cured in its early stages becomes fixed and incurable. Then the patient is to be supported for life. . . . Between the cost of supporting for a few months and that of supporting for life, no private economist, and certainly no political economist or statesman, should hesitate.[1]

The hospitals turned out to be economical because often they were mere barracks where the inmates subsisted on short rations and received little care—not curative therapies. The lack of concern, if not apathy, about the often dreadful conditions in mental institutions during the first part of this century is evidenced by the meager amounts of money allocated for them. When Jarvis submitted his *Report*, the average cost of maintaining a patient in a State hospital was $2.00 a week.[2] A century later, State hospitals were spending an average of $28 a week for the care of each patient. (Current costs in State hospitals range from $32 a day—in Mississippi—to $224 a day in Alaska.)[3] Although it is exceedingly difficult to make meaningful comparisons of dollar costs over a century, or even decades, the amount spent on State hospital patients was so low that the Joint Commission recommended in 1961 that the daily expenditure for each hospitalized patient should be tripled to about $12 a day during the next ten years. The Joint Commission recognized the need for treating patients within their own communities, but emphasized that the major portion of the recommended budget was to be allocated to the State hospitals. Thus, they held to the assumption that mental institutions were potentially beneficial, that perceived failures were the result of economic shortcomings that prevented them from functioning optimally, and that the remedy lay in greater funding to correct defects.

The Commission, however, could not have foreseen the sky-rocketing costs of hospitalization resulting in part from inflation and, perhaps to a greater degree, from technical and social factors that have disproportionately increased medical expenditures. So it is not only the assumed advantages of deinstitutional-ization, but also, the tremendously increased cost of operating State hospitals that have been responsible for closing many of them and moving patient care to the community sector. Federal funding of CMHCs and, later, of Medicare, Medicaid, and supplemental Social Security Insurance (SSI) programs gave the states an opportunity to shift much of the cost of caring for the mentally ill to the Federal Government.

The few available studies comparing the cost of care in the community with that in the hospital have yielded inconsistent findings. Weisbrod, Test, and Stein[4] carried out a cost-benefit comparison of patients hospitalized and given the usual follow-up treatment and of patients treated in an extensive community-based program in Wisconsin. Their well-conceptualized and thorough research with patients admitted to the hospital matched with those selected for community treatment showed that patient care was expensive in either setting—more than $7200 a year per patient. They reported that the total cost of the hospital-based program was "about 10% cheaper per patient" but that a con-sideration of all benefits and costs indicated that the community-based program provided some benefits to patients not supplied by the hospital-based program.

In 1976, Sharfstein and Nafziger[5] analyzed the costs of com-munity care over a three-year period for a middle-aged woman who had been hospitalized for eight years. The cost of care in the neighborhood health center decreased from $2100 in the first year to only $640 in the third, whereas costs in the alternative setting increased substantially.

In their 1976 cost-benefit analysis of community versus insti-tutional care, Murphy and Datel[6] projected an average saving of $20,800 for each community care patient over the next ten years. But that research is flawed because all Federal expenditures were not taken into account, revolving door patients were excluded, and the study lasted for only 8.5 months following discharge from the hospital.

Such limited, highly-selective studies do not allow for generalizations about the comparative costs of care in the community and in the hospital. In 1974, Robbins and Robbins[7] emphasized:

> Because the switch in emphasis to community programs did not include sufficient funding for research, there is no way to tell how many patients . . . are self-supporting or living on welfare at a lower cost than would have been the case had they remained in the hospital. However, for those who make use of the "revolving door," it may turn out that the annual costs for their care are considerably greater than if they had remained in the state hospital until they received the maximum therapeutic benefit. [*Quotes, ours.*]

There is no unanimity of opinion about the costs of properly maintaining chronic mental patients in the community. Reports of economic studies vary because line items used for computing costs differ widely. Quite possibly, community care for chronic patients is more expensive than care in comfortable state institutions. The costs of both hospital and community care have risen greatly because far-reaching economic forces, such as inflation and SSI programs, are involved. Precise costs in either setting are almost impossible to calculate because they include living expenses, loss of income for patients and sometimes family members, the financial burden to the family, and hidden expenses as well as the more direct cost of treatment.

In *summary*, without reliable data about comparative costs, a definite statement about the assumption that care in the community is less expensive than care in the hospital cannot be made at this time.

Care in the Community is Better Than Care in the Hospital

The widespread belief that care in the community (ideally in a family setting) was beneficial and desirable, in contrast to hospitalization which was considered potentially dehumanizing, encouraged the establishment of local mental health services and contributed substantially to deinstitutionalization. The first large wave of deinstitutionalized patients, during the years 1955 to 1969, appears to have been moderately well cared for in the community. Most patients were returned to family settings; only a minority went to community lodgings and agencies. But by the early and mid 1970s, the patients being "deinstitutionalized" tended to be a hard-core residual group who either had no families or communities or who had been hospitalized for so many years that they were now separated from former support systems. Segal notes:

> Each progressive cohort of returns to a mental hospital has a larger percentage of people in the cohort who have no family support or who have a limited amount of interaction with family members.[8]

During the last decade, therefore, many of the mentally ill have been housed in board-and-care or nursing homes where they are geographically located in the community but often not linked to any community support and care program. In their study of formerly hospitalized patients in California, aged 18 to 65, living in community-based sheltered care facilities, Segal and Aviram found that 52 percent had few or no relationships with family members; moreover, only 5 percent were married.[9] Advocates of deinstitutionalization seem to have grossly overestimated the familial and community support systems available to mental patients.

Maxwell Jones is representative of those who deplore the inadequacies of many of the community-based facilities. He states that many operators have had little or no training to enable them to care for mental patients and "with few exceptions, there is no planned program of activities." Jones concludes: "The tendency to use nursing and boarding homes cannot be equated with health planning, but rather with the lack of it."[10]

Evaluation of the assumption that community care is "better" than hospital care must be left to anecdote, bias, and opinion because we lack the data necessary to make informed statements about the comparative quality of care. We and many others have expressed concern about the variable quality of the care provided for chronic mental patients housed in nursing homes.[11] Possibly, the unregulated madhouses of the eighteenth century are being reincarnated in the efflorescence of nursing homes.

In *summary*, whether community care is better than hospital care is a question that is difficult to answer. The term "mental patient" is often used indiscriminately as if the mentally ill were a homogeneous rather than a heterogeneous group of people who have differing kinds of illnesses, needs, and resources. The limited research available has used differing methodologies and thus does not provide adequate comparisons on which judgment can be made about quality of care.

Comprehensive Care is a Desirable and Necessary Goal That Can Be Achieved in the Community

As mandated by Federal regulations, a CMHC must provide a comprehensive range of specific services in sufficient quantity to meet the needs of persons residing within the designated area.[12] As centers developed, however, many of them took license with the concept of comprehensiveness. For some centers, comprehensiveness meant a broad approach to a single illness, whereas others interpreted it to mean provision of needed services for all people in the area.[13]

Fueled by the enthusiasm of the Community Mental Health movement and the optimism of the "Great Society," the meaning of comprehensiveness expanded. For example, Reiman maintained that:

> A comprehensive community mental health program must concern itself not only with the mentally ill, but with the "well" population too— the 90% in need of practical mental health information and assistance.[14]

And, in 1964, Barton stated: "The ideal concept is that of a community health program that provides total mental health services to meet the total needs of the community."[15]

Regardless of the initial intent of the Federal regulations, comprehensiveness has been interpreted variably—according to the goals of a specific center. Many hospital- and university-based centers adhered to traditional approaches with "add-ons" to meet Federal requirements. In contrast, more "community-oriented" centers gave their priority to improvement of the quality of life in their catchment areas and tried to develop programs that psychiatry and other mental health disciplines had not heretofore offered. Some centers attempted to correct glaring defects in housing, employment, and education. When they recognized that such gains could be realized only by direct political activity, some centers joined in the "storming of the establishment."

During the 1960s, the Movement of Participatory Democracy and the Movement of Rising Expectations gave hope to the underprivileged.[16] CMHCs were organizations that communities expected to control through representative citizen participation. Governing boards were mandated; a majority of the members were to be from the catchment area. Many boards carried out their duties effectively but, especially in the earlier years, some became overinvolved in the promotion of political activities.

The implementation of comprehensive services was handicapped by Federal regulations that were initially intended to permit flexibility of operation but became more and more rigid and overloaded already burdened services with added requirements. As a result, bureaucratic inflexibility along with over-regulation limited the adaptability of some CMHCs and hindered their efforts to deliver comprehensive services. From the beginning, the Government tended to emphasize uniformity. Centers were forced into a Procrustean bed; the result was unworkable standardization.

The disastrous effects of releasing large numbers of chronic patients on unprepared communities and of discouraging admissions to hospitals has been described in GAP Report No. 102, THE CHRONIC MENTAL PATIENT IN THE COMMUNITY.[17] The State hospitals provided a total environment with an array of services that included: food and lodging, social contacts, opportunities to work, and entertainment, as well as treatment. The CMHCs found that it was difficult to offer or to supply these diverse services in the community, especially for chronically ill, socially disabled patients who have insufficient funds for even the necessities.

CMHCs compete with State hospitals for funds from the same "pot" and for the same community resources for patient placement. To lighten the burden of care for the seriously mentally ill, some CMHCs opted for the more glamorous and less taxing task of "preventing" mental illness. Thus, they enlarged the mental health system while not caring adequately for the chronically and the seriously ill.

In *summary*, comprehensiveness is an appealing assumption that was variably interpreted, at times so unrealistically that its implementation could not possibly be achieved. Furthermore, attempts to become comprehensive produced problems resulting from the overextension of mental health services. Limited resources and bureaucratic over-regulation further handicapped implementation efforts to the extent that comprehensive mental health services are more of a hope than a reality.

Continuity of Care is Beneficial

The fourth major assumption—that continuity of care is beneficial and could be achieved by centers—has its origin in both medical and social "womb-to-tomb" traditions. Without continuity, it is assumed that patients will not receive needed care and will regress; often the consequence is expensive, avoidable rehospitalization. However, continuity entails the risk of encouraging dependency. In practice, one must discriminate between efficient, necessary continuity and the needless dependency on the system.

Schwartz and Schwartz defined continuity of care as the "planning of a patient's treatment so that the help given at any point is part of a total program." [18] But continuity can also mean continuation of a relationship with the same organization, a relationship with the same helper, or the same help with different helpers. [19] Notwithstanding these differing views, the general idea that continuity—along with comprehensiveness—is beneficial became a powerful conceptual cornerstone of the Community Mental Health movement.

Wilder, Levin, and Zwerling posited that continuity must include treatment services, vocational rehabilitation services, and residential rehabilitation services. [20] Patients were to be provided with the appropriate type of care from the onset of illness through periods of decompensation to recovery. Recurrences were to be dealt with by a system sensitive to early indicators of mental distress, able to monitor patient progress, and ready to reinstitute care when needed. Care could be provided by a variety of appropriate specialists in the setting deemed most desirable and the coordinator would ensure continuity.

But in actuality, continuity of care is a complex concept. Bachrach has identified seven dimensions of continuity—longitudinality, individuality, comprehensiveness, flexibility, relationship, accessibility, and community. [21] It is exceedingly difficult to translate these dimensions of continuity into service delivery practices for many mental patients, especially the chronically ill, because of their special and costly, often life-long, service needs.

The large number of patients drawn into the CMHC network and the complexity of their problems generated a variety of programs in pursuit of the twin goals of continuity and comprehensiveness. Efforts to develop continuity of care called for linkage technology such as that described by Hansell. [22] Unitary record systems were created to keep track of patients' problems and treatment plans; the record would follow the patient through the various treatment settings within the system. The treatment team concept, developed in hospital milieus, became popular;

persons from various disciplines with differing skills joined to provide comprehensive care as a coordinated effort.[23]

But continuity of care within the CMHC was compromised by many problems. They included a deficiency in organizational technology, such territorial struggles as interdisciplinary rivalry, and an excessive demand for services that exceeded the capability of the system. The system could not adequately process the vast amounts of information about the large numbers of mentally ill. The problem-oriented record was not generally accepted and even where used, was not as helpful as anticipated.[24] Vitally-needed patient records could not be made readily available throughout the system and, without them, continuity was impossible.

Territorial issues were partially submerged in the initial enthusiasms for the CMHCs. But they surfaced after the early idealistic glow was diminished by the inherent frustrations of dealing with large numbers of patients who often presented refractory psychological dilemmas along with the problems of poverty. Collaboration among psychiatrists, psychologists, social workers, nurses, and paraprofessionals became strained. Psychiatrists reacted negatively to the ever-increasing power of their non-medical colleagues, to the reduction of their own roles, and to their loss of prestige.

But interdisciplinary rivalries were only one reason for the failure to achieve continuity of care. Conflicts also developed among the various components within the CMHCs. Territorial allegiance to one program, such as the outpatient clinic or the inpatient service, worked against the explicit CMHC policy that patients' needs should take precedence over those of the caregiving units. Intra-organizational fragmentation was particularly prevalent in centers lacking strong administrative leadership or in centers where the board and the staff became preoccupied with such social problems as racial bias, poverty, or poor housing.[25]

Efforts to achieve continuity of care were further hampered by conflicts among the CMHCs, State hospitals, and surrounding community agencies. Lack of interagency cooperation was the rule rather than the exception.

The volume of persons demanding services also hindered efforts to achieve continuity of care. The progressive deinstitutionalization of hospital patients and the flow of large numbers of chronic patients into the community further overloaded the system. The numbers of patients referred from the State hospitals and actually returning to CMHCs to receive followup care—just one link in the system—have been extremely variable. Many CMHCs had to struggle just to keep pace with the emergent and most obvious problems. Continuity of care received a low priority.

Continuity of care is a cherished, highly-valued core concept in both community mental health and health care generally. But the concept has been variously defined and there have been few adequate studies of its implementation.[26]

For continuity of care to be achieved, priorities must be established; unfortunately, many centers never effectively set priorities. The numerous problems encountered by centers made it very difficult for them even to attempt to offer continuity of care. Centers cannot provide continuity when they are overloaded by demands for services and constrained by the inflexibility of Federal over-regulation. Other problems hindering them from providing continuity of care were: intra-agency and interagency rivalries and conflicts, lack of funding for coordination of services, and a scarcity of resources. It appears that the vigorous advocates of continuity of care failed to recognize the impediments to continuity produced by the immensity and the complexity of chronic mental illness. The lack of well-designed studies of continuity makes it impossible for us to assess its validity scientifically.

In *summary*, continuity of care is an attractive assumption that appears to have *prima facie* validity. But there have been serious problems with definition and implementation of continuity and there has been little research on it.

The Designation of Catchment Areas Enhances the Provision of Services

The 1963 CMHC Act required each state to be divided into catchment areas containing 75,000 to 200,000 persons before any CMHC could be established. Foley described how the term "community" was defined.

> We came down to simply "numbers of people because other approaches— political, geographic, ethnic, or socioeconomic boundaries—did not work. Quantities of population was the last resort.[27]

This "numerical" decision has produced major problems. Perhaps the first and foremost has been the confounding of a catchment area with the traditional concept of a community. In "The Concept of Community: The Short Circuit of the Mental Health Movement," Panzetta states that the "movement has glorified the concept of community without adequately understanding it."[28] At least implicitly, the catchment area was intended to provide patients with a caring social network, a characteristic of *Gemeinschaft* communities where social life is maintained by common customs, shared sentiments, and active participation of the entire society in matters affecting the welfare of the inhabitants. What was overlooked was that these community characteristics must be present or most arise organically and cannot be superimposed on a group of people or artificially produced by the mere designation of the area according to the number of its residents. Many critics believe that the CMHC is still searching for a community.

The assumption that geographic responsibility was necessary to insure that needed services would be provided to all persons in a designated area sprang from Public Health successes with geographic districts. It was believed that defined geographic areas of responsibility would improve quality of care and enhance accessibility and availability of services.[29] Later, other advantages were enumerated: the catchment area would foster continuity of care, decrease the barriers to care, make gaps in services obvious, promote the development of smaller units than had existed in State facilities, and enable the public to know more about the community and community agencies.

The second problem was created by the arbitrary definition of the size of the population to be served without regard for either population density or geographic considerations. In both populous urban and sparsely-settled rural areas, the population requirement seemed to be rigid and often self-defeating. For instance, merely because its designated population of 741,324 (1960) did not conform to Federal specification, the NIMH turned down Milwaukee's proposal to have one central facility and six neighborhood teams. Some who administered services in highly disorganized and fractious urban areas suggested that 25,000 persons might be the optimal number to be served in their communities.[30] And some rural areas with widely dispersed populations advocated abandoning the rigid numerical requirements altogether.[31]

A few months after passage of the CMHC legislation, a publication of the Joint Information Service described eleven examples of community mental health services to illustrate the current state of the art and to provide models for future efforts.[32] Four had no service areas and seven served populations ranging from 93,000 to one million persons. In retrospect, it is ironic to note that the largest was the CMHC in Ft. Logan, Colorado, which has often been held to be "the" model, even though the number of people within it far exceeds Federal guidelines. In 1968, the populations of various catchment areas ranged in size from 39,000 to 256,000; fully 10 percent of funded Federal CMHCs were at variance with the standards.[33]

A third problem stemmed from the imposition of arbitrary geographic boundaries rather than the use of natural ecologic borders or existing political and service districts. In some large metropolitan areas already subdivided and complicated by over-lapping jurisdictions, the imposition of the new catchment areas that coincided with no existing service or political boundaries further fragmented the delivery of human services. The realities of everyday life—established transportation, work, communication, and health service patterns—were disregarded.

Fourth, it was often difficult to obtain political and economic support for these arbitrarily defined catchment areas. Many did not coincide with political subdivisions and thus were cut off from the political and economic base for most human services. Such lack of local budgetary support led to grievous problems.

Fifth, the new catchment areas produced problems for certain special groups. Whereas some politically powerful constituencies successfully pressured centers for services, many small groups lacked either a sufficient critical mass or the political clout to get the attention they needed. For example, the mentally ill who also belonged to such small subgroups as the blind, deaf, or retarded were often underserved.

In theory, catchment areas were established to insure geographic responsibility. In practice, this arrangement led to denial of services, buck-passing, and even the falsification of addresses, especially in those areas hard pressed to provide comprehensive services for disorganized neighborhoods.[34]

Despite these serious problems, there have been only a few thorough studies of the influence of the catchment area design on the provision and utilization of mental health services.[35] A national study in 1972 showed that there were greater resources in catchment areas served by CMHCs than in catchment areas without CMHCs.[36] This finding, however, reveals more about the resources in such areas than about the catchment area concept. Although there have been serious problems with delineating boundaries, an Arthur D. Little study reported that the catchment area served by a CMHC than by a control population reported a much greater utilization of services by residents of a catchment area served by a CMHC than be a control population from a "dummy" catchment area served by a multiservice center. They concluded that catchment areas increased utilization of mental health services and, therefore, that CMHCs could fulfill the mandate to provide comprehensive and coordinated mental health care for the residents of geographically-defined areas.

Although the concept of the catchment area appears to have validity to the extent that it defines the area of service responsibility, faulty implementation produced serious difficulties in many places. The essential flaw was the early decision to relate the size of the catchment area solely to numbers of people without regard for either existing political and geographic boundaries or for the realities of everyday life for the average person. What was intended to be a transfer of services and people from institutions to the community became a transfer to the catchment area. But community and catchment area are not synonymous. As Huffine and Craig[39] assert, the inhabitants of a catchment area may or may not constitute a community or even several communities.

The 1980 Mental Health Systems Act calls for abandoning the term "catchment area" and replacing it with the designation, "mental health service area."[40] The changed terminology may diminish semantic confusion but does little to simplify the serious problems produced by the initial decision to define such areas arbitrarily—merely by numbers of people.

In *summary*, the availability of mental health services for all in a defined area who need them is a desirable goal and the catchment area design was established to enable CMHCs to meet that goal. In its implementation, however, it encountered formidable handicaps because mental health services were tied to geographic areas that had neither political nor natural boundaries, that disregarded fixed patterns of everyday existence, that neglected special populations, and that did not have the flexibility necessary to give services either to densely packed or to sparsely inhabited areas.

Accessibility to Mental Health Services is Essential

Accessibility was deemed necessary because of the relative isolation of many public mental hospitals and the existing barriers to private psychiatric care. The "asylum" concept had held that a sheltered, bucolic environment was salutary; consequently, many older public hospitals were built in rural or small town settings where land was relatively inexpensive. As a result, hospitalized patients were separated from their families and from other natural support systems. Furthermore, the relative isolation made it difficult for the hospitals to attract and retain professional staffs.

In addition to the geographic barriers, other factors limited the access of large segments of the population to psychiatric care. Private psychiatric treatment was not only costly but also was effectively reserved for patients considered to be appropriate for certain types of treatment. The mal-distribution of professionals increased the problems of accessibility. During the first half of this century the ascendancy of psychoanalysis influenced many psychiatrists to adopt a psychotherapeutic model of practice which excluded many of the mentally ill because they did not fit the criteria for "good" psychotherapy patients. Also, many psychiatrists in private practice often did not treat children, the elderly, members of minority groups, the minimally educated, the poor, or the chronically ill. Furthermore, practitioners tended to congregate in heavily populated areas where there was a large potential pool of patients seeking psychotherapy, an opportunity to associate with kindred professionals, and the presence of many cultural attractions. The result was a severe mal-distribution of psychiatrists.

In order to receive Federal funding, the centers initially were required to make an array of services accessible to the public. Some centers found ingenious ways to make these services accessible. For example, in 1965, the Lincoln Hospital Center in the South Bronx established neighborhood "store front" centers, each serving 23,000 people in five square blocks.[41] In 1967, the West Philadelphia Center established satellites in each of its seven different ethnic, economic, and cultural neighborhoods.[42] A NIMH document reported that some CMHCs in rural areas also were establishing small satellite clinics distant from the central installation.[43]

Outreach became highly fashionable as centers discovered that many catchment area residents were uninformed about psychosocial problems or reluctant to seek help for them. Centers advertised to inform the public about their services and locations. It was hoped that an interagency network would promote easy referral of patients from one agency to another. Many outreach offices opened "walk-in" services that did away with the usual intake procedures and waiting lists. A nonexclusion policy was fostered and instant help was guaranteed to anyone coming through the door.

There have been major problems with accessibility. The first is fiscal. With increasing costs and decreasing Federal support, many CMHCs have attempted to become cost-effective by curtailing services that do not produce revenue and by giving priority to those that do. For example, costly, time-consuming services such as home visits to indigent patients have been reduced in favor of office hours for paying patients; consultations often are provided only to agencies able to pay for them. Also, increased dependence on Medicaid and Medicare payments has prompted many CMHCs to alter their programs so that they can receive such funds.

A second problem is presented by non-English speaking minority groups. For example, the Census Bureau estimates that Hispanic-Americans will be the largest minority in the United States within a few years.[44] Providing adequate mental health services for them necessitates more than attention to their symptoms. It requires a bilingual staff and awareness of the problems of acculturation and of culture conflict.

Difficulties in supplying services to rural areas is a third problem of accessibility. In many rural catchment areas that exceed 5,000 square miles, their geographically isolated centers are underutilized. Lack of transportation, bad weather conditions, and the time lost from work by family members and patients are all seen as realistic barriers to care. However, comparative rural-urban utilization studies report that the most significant factors limiting the use of centers in rural areas are lack of awareness and understanding about the available services and fear of stigmatization.[45]

There is a severe lack of services and professional personnel in rural America. Compared to urban areas, including those with large numbers of poor people, many rural areas are understaffed and have the least comprehensive service patterns of any centers. Additional problems include inadequate transportation and unavailability of 24-hour services. All of these problems are compounded when the rural area is also a poverty area.[46]

Lack of accessibility and availability of services seem to have been less troublesome problems to CMHCs than difficulties with administration, funding, and manpower distribution or the development of truly viable services for neglected populations— the poor, children, the elderly, substance abusers, and the chronically ill. A recent survey solicited the opinions of 390 CMHC directors and public mental hospital directors on the critical issues for community mental health. Of fifty-seven issues ranked according to priority, the only one relating to accessibility—the need for a greater outreach effort—was twenty-fourth.

In *summary,* there are complex fiscal and attitudinal as well as geographic barriers limiting accessibility. These difficulties coupled with the shortage of professionals, with arbitrary and unrealistic catchment area boundaries, and with bureaucratic inflexibilities have made accessibility an ideal that has not yet been realized.

The Social Environment Produces Mental Illness

Prior to the passage of the CMHC Act of 1963, it was increasingly believed that the social environment was the locus for the cause and hence the treatment of mental illness. This belief was shaped by:

- American pragmatism and the "can do" attitude which were especially strong after World War II. Many psychiatrists believed that with an all-out effort and the utilization of our immense resources we could control mental illness. Influenced by Adolf Meyer's concept of mental illness as a reaction to adversity, social psychiatry emerged as a special field of interest.
- The idea that human nature was socially determined.[47] Some social scientists argued that mental illness was a condition that could be explained and treated as a type of deviance from the social norm.[48]
- The early "anti-psychiatry" movement which stated that society and psychiatrists "produced" mental illness. According to Szasz,[49] labeling an individual as "sick reflected society's prejudices and treating disturbed behavior as an illness was a form of oppression.
- The finding that family factors, such as the double bind, or pseudomutuality, played an important role in the etiology of schizophrenia was misinterpreted to mean that they were the sole cause.[50, 51] It followed that interventions directed toward the environment (family) would alleviate or prevent mental disorder.
- The results of community studies in New Haven, Stirling County, and Midtown Manhattan showing that adverse social conditions were correlated with both the frequency of mental illness and the type of treatment received (if any).[52–57]

Thus, the social environment was seen as potentially noxious and mental institutions as sinister. Goffman's[58] description of the heretofore little known "underside" of State hospital life heightened the contradictions between custody and treatment. In his view, State hospitals tended to foster rather than cure "pathological" behavior. A core of politically-minded psychiatrists became convinced that community psychiatry—by this time almost indistinguishable from the Community Mental Health movement—not only would offer more humane and effective therapies than institutions, but also could successfully attack the causes of mental illness in the social environment.

When the Joint Commission recommended an extension of the State hospital system, Robert Felix, the Director of the NIMH, disagreed, saying: "Considerably more attention could have been placed upon steps aimed at prevention of mental illness and upon maintenance of mental health in the development of a 'National Action' program." [59]

"Maintenance" of mental health became synonymous with environmental manipulation. With the advent of the New Frontier, Congressional legislation committed the Federal Government to mental health programs and an attack upon the presumed causes of mental illness. Although President Kennedy realized that further research was needed to find a cure for mental illness, he stated that:

> The general strengthening of our fundamental community, social welfare,and educational programs can do much to eliminate or correct the harsh environmental conditions which often are associated with mental retardation and mental illness. [60]

Many psychiatrists jumped on the CMHC bandwagon. For example, Leonard Duhl wrote:

> We are in fact building a program which is to be concerned with all aspects of the prevention, care, and treatment of the mentally ill, as well as the critical institutions which play a role in the normal development of the individual in the care and treatment of disease. [61]

Gerald Caplan recommended that the psychiatric consultant learn to intervene on the patient's behalf at the group or institutional level. Then, "gradually more and more cases are handled within the social system of the organization without referral and even without consultation." [62] The final step for the psychiatrist is to become:

an advisor on general institutional action . . . to exercise the most potent preventive and remedial influence on large numbers of actual or potential sufferers among the firm's members.[63]

Some psychiatrists in the vanguard of those attempting to improve the social environment advocated that psychiatrists become political activists.[64] In his critique, "Radical Psychiatry: An Examination of the Issues," Talbott cited psychiatrists who "emphasized that their task should be political involvement and social change rather than intrapsychic change."[65] Perhaps the most far-reaching scheme was proposed by Arsenian who recommended social engineering on a grand scale as the solution to all psychological problems.[66]

Zusman described sociological approaches which dealt with mental illness as deviance. He predicted that, with the incorporation of the deviant mentally ill into the mainstream,

most mental hospitals and prisons as we presently know them may disappear to become an administrative office which controls the whereabouts and treatment activities of scattered patients or prisoners.[67]

How much time was actually spent in "treating" the environment is not easy to determine. Ozarin[68] states that in 1974, only 5.7 percent of all CMHC's staff hours were allocated to extramural consultation whereas 4.5 percent of the extramural time was case oriented. Case reports[69] emphasized involvement with community organizations; primary goals were to "modify features of the social, economic, and institutional environment that breed alienation, apathy, regression, and powerlessness."[70]

In 1965, Dunham[71] described flaws in the assumption that the social environment produced mental illness and predicted that CMHCs would soon encounter serious difficulties for the following reasons:

- There was no evidence to indicate that working at the community level to treat mental patients was effective.

- Attempting to use community-level techniques to reduce mental disturbances was "likely to remove the psychiatrist still further from the more *bona fide* cases of mental illness." [72]
- Even if the psychiatrist had a role within the CMHC power structure, his or her professional effectiveness would be reduced. [73]
- Psychiatrists would be "pushed in a direction not entirely of their own making" and subjected to a blurring of their professional roles and identity. [74]

Unfortunately, many of the problems foreseen by Dunham have become realities. First, it has not been demonstrated that community[75] organization can improve mental health within the community. Second, the *"bona fide* ill" have been seriously neglected. In 1978, Bachrach wrote:

> Community mental health planning is *de facto* geared toward care of persons who can, for the most part and most of the time, look after themselves. [76]

In the CMHCs, schizophrenics constituted only 12 percent and alcoholics only 8 percent of the case load. [77] Talbott[78] cites a study which estimated that adequate aftercare is provided for only 25 percent of chronic mental patients. But we should realize that psychiatrists in private practice also have neglected this population; schizophrenics make up only 11.3 percent of all office visits to all psychiatrists whereas those with neuroses, personality disorders, transitional disorders, or vague complaints make up 66.2 percent. [79]

Dunham's third and fourth predictions—that the effectiveness of psychiatrsits in CMHCs would be reduced and that their role would be blurred—have materialized. It appears that the psychiatrists' roles in the CMHC have diminished. Often medical staff are limited to writing prescriptions and seeing patients in the least possible time necessary to obtain Medicaid payments.

CMHCs have had a steadily decreasing population of psychiatrists on their staffs.[80] The percentage of directors who are psychiatrists dropped from 55 percent in 1971 to 26 percent in 1977.[81] Borus notes that psychiatrists:

> deceived themselves into trying to fulfill the public illusion that psychiatry could solve societal problems, . . . public disillusionment with CMH followed shortly thereafter when the impossible could not be delivered.[82]

In a retrospective view of what he called the "heroic phase" of community psychiatry, Bellak stated:

> a liberal ideology facilitated the desire to extend care for mental health to include help with the problems of an economic, social and cultural nature.[83]

This ideology has had some beneficial effects; it stimulated refinements in the research on social and family dimensions of mental illness and led to the development of social approaches to rehabilitation.[84–86] But the CMHC program has been costly— not only in dollars but also in the resulting disillusionment and lost opportunities. Zusman emphasizes that:

> scarce professional resources and energy [have been diverted] from direct treatment, much of whose value is clearly demonstrable, into work in the community where the professionals have only limited expertise and where there is no evidence that their work can have any effect on mental illness or on the function of a mental health center.[87]

Along with the emerging conservatism of America in the early 1980s, as evidenced by drastic reductions in funding for social programs and psychiatry's current enthusiasm for biological research, we are observing less national concern about the significance of social factors in the etiology and treatment of mental illness and even about the quality of the social environment.

In *summary,* the complexity of the social environment was underestimated and the thesis that the social environment produces mental illness was overemphasized. As a result, goals became diffuse, roles became blurred, and the most seriously ill were not given the high priority for service they needed. Environmental stressors can be precipitants of mental illness and social factors can influence its cause, course, and treatment, although they may not be central to its etiology. But there is no scientific evidence to support the assumption that "treating" the social environment will diminish the incidence of mental illness. Focusing mental health efforts on improving the social environment is unrealistically expensive; such efforts dilute already scarce human and material resources. Heavy involvement in community action programs destroyed the clinical effectiveness of some CMHCs.

Preventive Efforts Can Reduce the Incidence and Prevalence of Mental Illnesses

Although definitions of community psychiatry vary somewhat, they generally include the responsibility to reduce the number of mentally ill within a given population.[88] In this respect, community psychiatry is closely related to public health which seeks to prevent potential or actual health problems through systematic action.[89] Community psychiatry has advocated the public health approach to mental illness, particularly the application of principles of primary prevention. By definition, primary prevention consists of measures taken for people whose health is good although they may belong to a "population at risk." In psychiatry it is a relatively recent concept.

Primary prevention needs to justify the diversion of public funds from the treatment and care of the mentally ill to preventive action by furnishing proof that lessened morbidity will result. Currently, lack of such evidence has made primary prevention a controversial issue although it continues to be an attractive concept. The mentally ill could be better served if the number of new cases could be contained; demands for services always seem to outstrip available human and material resources.

Scientific efforts to prevent mental illness antedate the development of CMHC programs. The assumption that mental illnesses were manifestations of organic conditions had validity for general paresis and for psychosis accompanying pellagra. These once common diseases are now rare because preventive measures have been effective. At the beginning of this century, efforts were made to reduce mental illnesses by eugenics and by controlling immigration. One-half century prior to the CMHC legislation, the Mental Hygiene Movement called for prompt detection and control of unhealthy conditions, establishment of a network of community services, and public education. But there was little public support for community programs aimed at the prevention of mental illnesses until their high prevalence was recognized during World War II.

The Joint Commission warned only a few years later that the Mental Hygiene Movement's emphasis on prevention had diverted attention from the major mental disorders.

> A National Health Program should avoid the risk of false promise in "education for better mental health" and focus on the more modest goal of disseminating such information about mental illness as the public needs and wants in order to recognize psychological forms of sickness and to strive at an informed opinion of its responsibility toward the mentally ill.[90]

Such warnings went unheeded. Instead, the nation was inclined to follow President Kennedy's stirring 1963 message, "Prevention should be given highest priority..."[91] Some preventive concepts had already been developed. Erich Lindemann[92] had proposed principles of crisis intervention and he and his associates had supplied a conceptual framework for preventive psychiatry. The Grant Foundation had supported a commission to prepare for the 5th International Congress of Child Psychiatry at Scheveningen, Holland in 1962—the first international meeting devoted entirely to the primary prevention of mental disorders in children.[93]

Many psychiatrists indulged in optimistic expectations—the

age of preventive psychiatry had arrived. They persuaded policy makers to emphasize prevention in new mental health legislation. But only a few psychiatrists had training in public health even though some schools of public health had included mental health issues in their curricula for many years. In the 1960s, preventive programs in psychiatry often resembled social reform programs; they reflected the spirit of the times and were linked more to the War on Poverty and to the Civil Rights movement than to psychiatry.

In 1964, the Federal Government attempted to persuade psychiatrists to "accept the challenge of providing leadership in community mental health programs."[94] Four regional training institutes in community psychiatry brought together educators from many psychiatric departments to develop new guidelines for the psychiatrist's professional role. Raymond Feldman, Deputy Director of NIMH, stated:

> The broad dimensions of community mental health pose a distinct challenge for psychiatrists. . . . psychiatry has no real alternative to active, intelligent participation in the future unfolding of events.[95]

About the same time, Caplan's *Principles of Preventive Psychiatry*[96] was hailed as a:

> Bible [which] should be read by every psychiatric resident and mental health worker in training as well as by those who are engaged in community mental health programs.[97]

Caplan[98] suggested a two-level conceptual model for primary prevention that intentionally overemphasized environmental factors because the etiology of major mental disorders was largely unknown. He assumed that mental health could be promoted and mental illness thereby reduced by: (1) insuring the availability of physical, psychosocial, and sociocultural supplies; and (2) enabling people to cope successfully with crises—the recurrent changes in life situations that upset the customary equilibrium and can lead to decompensation.

The primary prevention programs instituted by some centers, however, often appeared to be no more than public relations projects. There was little scientific evidence to support the desirability of, or the necessity for, primary prevention programs and the failure of centers to conduct evaluation research further weakened the belief that such programs were worthwhile. Many CMHCs made only token efforts to comply with Federal demands for primary prevention programs perhaps, in part, because they usually did not produce revenue. Some CMHCs consider crisis intervention to be a form of primary prevention and others restrict their preventions programs to a "hotline."

Zusman presents the somewhat pessimistic views of primary prevention held by many psychiatrists today. He considers "inadequate definitions of terms and lack of research" the greatest weakness in primary prevention.[99] In the same vein, after reviewing sixty studies of efforts to improve mental health, Davis concluded that "so-called principles of mental hygiene are vague slogans rather than strategies of behavior which can be put into practice," that advice is ineffective, and that there is no known preventive measure for the major psychoses at this time.[100] In essence, mental health educators have little or nothing specific and practical to tell the public.

Much of the criticism of primary prevention appears to be justified and may explain the current slackening of professional interest in it. These criticisms, however, may be too harsh and may underestimate the continuing need to explore ways to improve the general conditions of life and thereby reduce human misery. Notwithstanding widespread skepticism, continuing concern led the President's Commission on Mental Health to convene a Task Panel on Prevention. In its April 1979 Report,[101] the Commission emphasized the need for continued efforts toward primary prevention. Significantly, five of the eight recommendations advocated attention to and better care for children as the most desirable preventive measure.

An HEW Task Force established to respond to the Report of

the President's Commission on Mental Health reacted skeptically to the Task Panel's challenge[102] to develop strategies which effectively reduce the incidence of mental illness in large populations at a feasible cost. The Task Force stated:

> Without a broad understanding of the etiology of psychopathology—plus a plan to identify specific antecedents and concomitants of mental and emotional problems—the expenditure of funds may not move us closer to preventing mental illness than we are now.[103]

In *summary,* primary prevention is an appealing assumption but there is little evidence for its validity. The emphasis on primary prevention has led to a neglect of the two tertiary prevention programs, rehabilitation and aftercare, which were not even included among the five essential services in the original legislation. Also, the belief in primary prevention has led to a disregard for disease models which were seen as irrelevant to mental illness.

Local Responsibility and Control are Necessary to Insure the Success of CMHCs

The CMHC program began at a time when people across the nation were striving for increased personal control of their lives, services, and government. Parallel developments in civil rights, education, and local control of government provided the setting for community participation in mental health. This new individualism and the drive for local self-determination can be seen as reactions to the increasing centralization of Federal and State authority that followed the anti-Depression and World War II efforts. The ninth assumption of the CMHC planners, therefore, was that it was necessary for the local community to assume responsibility for, and control of, the services provided.

The rationale for local responsibility and control was based on the belief that the citizenry would forge a new partnership with professionals to identify, plan, and meet the mental health needs of the community. Also, it stemmed from the conviction that bottom-up planning and program development could be tailored to the special and often specific needs of a local community. It was believed that organizing the community for needs assessments and other programs would improve the services delivered. Community involvement would facilitate funding, establish true priorities of services, increase acceptance of services in the community, and would alter attitudes and prejudices toward mental illness.

Local control was implemented by the CMHC Act of 1963 which mandated the creation of citizen boards and by the enabling legislation passed by most states in the mid-1960s which gave advisory and other control functions to local communities. The National Mental Health Association and its chapters, other organizations, and various former patient, self-help, and advocacy groups developed a constituency favoring community control of CMHCs. Insistence on local citizens' boards for Federally-funded CMHCs shifted the governance and fiscal responsibility toward the community.

But the implementation of local responsibility and control in CMHCs has been spotty despite the Federal funding of over 750 Centers. Some CMHCs have enjoyed community participation and partnerships with providers; a few have gone the route of real community control; others have weak or minimal to non-existent community participation. Although the responses of some communities to the needs of unserved and underserved populations have been dramatic and rewarding, in many communities there has been frustration, disappointment, or apathy about mental illness.

Major difficulties with local responsibility concern such issues as: (1) an insufficient number of qualified, interested, and committed citizens; (2) the usurpation of power by cliques; (3) conflicts among various interest groups; and (4) ambiguity concerning who is in control and over what? Furthermore, Federal and

State commitments to local control and to bottom-up planning sometimes conflict with mandated Federal or State fiscal and program priorities and also with local concerns and priorities. Local priorities frequently have disregarded or led to the exclusion of the most severely and chronically mentally ill patients.

Another major problem is that State and Federal time frames for plans, budgets, and priorities frequently do not allow for adequate local input. Broad State or Federal mandates are often distorted and misinterpreted at the local level, contributing to a further breakdown of communication and lack of trust. Perhaps the most serious problem arises when there is no consensus about control or about fiscal or service priorities. Ugly battles ensue. Who is really in control? Unfortunately, the needs of the people, especially of the severely and chronically ill, are lost in political battles over prerogatives and territory.

Nationally, community control is uneven; it works well and meets needs in some places but is almost nonexistent in others. Tensions exist because of conflicts about program priorities, control, and funding.

CMHCs appear to work most effectively where: (1) there is a real partnership between citizens and providers; (2) the citizens are well trained and motivated; (3) there is mutual respect between providers and recipients of care; and (4) there is a genuine concern about those in greatest need. In CMHCs enjoying moderate success there are problems with negotiation and consensus. Those CMHCs with serious problems are characterized by: (1) a lack of relationships and negotiation; (2) entrenched citizen or professional groups; (3) stereotyping on both sides; (4) little focus on the needs of the people to be served; and (5) controversies over territory and power.

The need to have community involvement in planning, developing, and monitoring mental health programs is basically a sound assumption. In practice, it must be accompanied by reminders to give the highest priority for services to those in greatest need and the unserved. The day is long past when professionals alone can speak for the needs of the community. For years, lay boards of trustees for hospitals and clinics have identified needs and worked for quality health care in partnership with professionals. In CMHCs, community participation is necessary to assure that the professionals recognize and meet the needs defined by the community. Otherwise, services become divorced from both the needs of the population and the frames of reference that have meaning for the community.

The change in taxation during the last twenty years has diminished local fiscal resources. In 1976, 66 percent of the tax dollar went to the Federal Government, 18 percent to State Governments, and 16 percent to local governments whereas twenty years previously, the percentages were almost reversed—the local and State Governments obtained the major portion of the tax dollar. We should recall that during the 1930s there was widespread disillusionment with the capabilities of local communities; the bright young people went to work for the Federal Government because they had opportunities to develop plans and programs that might "cure" the Depression. But in the last two decades, the pendulum has swung back to local rather than Federal control. This major political shift, dramatized by the 1980 election, indicates implicitly and explicitly that states and communities will have to control, fund, and be responsible for their own mental health programs.

In *summary*, attempts to implement local control often produced problems. Federal guidelines for local control were based on naive beliefs about the willingness and expertise of most communities. Moreover, it was taken for granted that communities had resources; in reality, many had few. Too often, there was "top-down" not "bottom-up" planning. The many problems with implementation have made it impossible to evaluate scientifically the assumption that local control is necessary to ensure the success of the CMHCs.

REFERENCES

1. See citation 1, Chapter 2.
2. Ibid.
3. Personal communication with the Clearinghouse, NIMH, 20 April 1981.
4. Weisbrod, B. A., M. A. Test, and L. I. Stein. Alternative mental hospital treatment: II: Economic benefit cost-analysis, *Archives of General Psychiatry*, 37(4):400–405, 1980.
5. Sharfstein, S. S., and J. C. Nafziger. Community care: Costs and benefits for a chronic patient, *Hospital & Community Psychiatry*, 37(3):171–176, 1976.
6. Murphy, J. G., and W. E. Datel. A cost-benefit analysis of community versus institutional living, *Hospital & Community Psychiatry*, 27(3):165–179, 1976.
7. Robbins, E., and L. Robbins. Charge to the community: Some early effects of a State Hospital system's change of policy, *American Journal of Psychiatry*, 131(6):641–645, 1974.
8. Segal, S. P. Community care and deinstitutionalization: A review, *Social Work*, 24(6):521–527, 1974.
9. _____, and U. Aviram. Community-based sheltered care. In *State Mental Hospitals: What Happens When They Close?* P. I. Ahmed and S. C. Plog (Eds.). New York: Plenum Publishing Corp., 1976, pp. 111–124.
10. Jones, M. Community care for chronic mental patients: The need for reassessment, *Hospital & Community Psychiatry*, 26(2):94–98, 1975.
11. Group for the Advancement of Psychiatry. Committee on Psychiatry and the Community. *The Chronic Mental Patient in the Community*. Report No. 102. New York: Mental Health Materials Center, Inc., 1978.
12. *Federal Register*. Washington, DC: USGPO, May, 1964.
13. See citation 4.
14. Reiman, D. *Mental Health in the Community Public Health Program*. Austin, TX: Hogg Foundation for Mental Health, 1962.
15. Barton, W. E. Quoted in citation 25, Chapter 2.

16. Steenfeldt-Foss, O. Elements of a comprehensive psychiatric service, *Southern Psychiatric Quarterly,* 48(4):14–17, 1974.
17. See citation 11, pp. 277–280.
18. Schwartz, M. S., and C. B. Schwartz. *Social Approaches to Mental Care.* New York: Columbia University Press, 1974.
19. Ibid., p. 171.
20. Wilder, J. F., G. Levin, and I. Zwerling. Planning and developing the locus of care. In *The Practice of Community Mental Health,* H. Grunebaum (Ed.). Boston: Little Brown & Company, 1970.
21. Bachrach, L. L. Continuity of care for chronic mental patients: A conceptual analysis, *American Journal of Psychiatry,* 138:1449–1456, 1981.
22. Hansell, N. Services for schizophrenics: A lifelong approach to treatment, *Hospital & Community Psychiatry,* 29:105–109, 1978.
23. Test, M. A. Continuity of care in community treatment, *New Directions in Mental Health Services,* 2:15–23, 1979.
24. Panzetta, A. F. The concept of the community: The short-circuit of the mental health movement, *Archives of General Psychiatry,* 25:291–297, 1971.
25. Ibid.
26. See citation 21.
27. Foley, H. *Community Mental Health Legislation: The Formative Process.* Lexington, MA: Lexington Books, 1975.
28. See citation 24.
29. Weston, W. D. Development of community mental health concepts. In *Comprehensive Textbook of Psychiatry,* A. M. Freedman, H. I. Kaplan, and B. J. Sadock (Eds.). Vol. II. Baltimore: Williams and Wilkins, 1975, pp. 2310–2322.
30. Kaplan, S. "The Use and Abuse of Federal Derived Health Delivery Funds as Instruments of Political Action: The Lincoln Hospital Mental Health Center." Unpublished manuscript.
31. *Report of the President's Commission on Mental Health: Task Panel on Rural Mental Health.* Vol. 3. Washington, DC: USGPO, 1978, pp. 1155–1190.
32. Glasscote, R. M., J. N. Sussex, E. Cumming, and L. H. Smith. *The Community Mental Health Center: An Interim Appraisal.* Washington, DC: Joint Information Center Service, 1969.

33. See citation 25, Chapter 2.
34. Regester, D. C. Community mental health—for whose community? *American Journal of Public Health*, 64:886–893, 1974.
35. Ozarin, L. D. Community mental health: Does it work? Review of the evaluation literature. See citation 4, Chapter 2.
36. National Study Service. *Relative Impact of Various Factors in the Development of Mental Health Resources.* Contract HSM 42-70-108. January 1972.
37. *Viability of the Catchment Area.* Contract HSM 42-72-96. Cambridge, MA: Arthur D. Little Co., 1973.
38. Tischler, G. L., J. Henisz, J. K. Myers, and V. Garrison. The impact of catchmenting, *Administration of Mental Health*, 1:22–29, 1972.
39. Huffine, C. L., and T. J. Craig. Catchment and community, *Archives of General Psychiatry*, 28:483–488, 1973.
40. See citation 67, Chapter 2.
41. Lasch, C. *Haven in a Heartless World.* New York: Basic Books, Inc., 1977.
42. Bateson, G., D. D. Jackson, H. Hale, and J. H. Weakland. Toward a theory of schizophrenia, *Behavioral Science*, 1:251–264, 1956.
43. *The Mental Health of Rural America: The Rural Programs of the National Institute of Mental Health*, J. Segal (Ed.). Rockville, MD: NIMH, 1973.
44. Personal communication, U.S. Bureau of the Census, April, 1982.
45. Bachrach, L. L. *Human Services in Rural Areas: An Analytical Review.* Human Services Monograph Series No. 21. Rockville, MD: Project Share, June, 1981.
46. Ibid.
47. Seely, J. R. Social values: The mental health movement and mental health, *American Academy of Political and Social Science*, 286:15–24, 1953.
48. See citation 41.
49. Szasz, T. *The Myth of Mental Illness: Foundation of a Theory of Personal Conduct.* New York: Dell, 1961.
50. See citation 42.
51. Wynne, L. C., I. M. Ryckoh, J. Day, and S. Hirsch. Pseudomutuality on the family relations of schizophrenics, *Psychiatry*, 21:205–220, 1958.
52. See citation 45, Chapter 2.

53. See citation 47, Chapter 2.

54. Hughes, C. C., A. M. Tremblay, R. N. Rapoport, and A. H. Leighton. *People of Cove and Woodlot.* New York: Basic Books, Inc., 1960.

55. Leighton, D. C., J. S. Harding, D. B. Macklin, A. M. Macmillan, and A. H. Leighton. *The Character of Danger.* New York: Basic Books, Inc., 1963.

56. See citation 49, Chapter 2.

57. Langner, T. S., and S. T. Michael. *Life Stress and Mental Health.* Vol. II of the Midtown Manhattan Study Thomas A. C. Rennie Series in Social Psychiatry. Glencoe, IL: The Free Press of Glencoe, 1963.

58. See citation 48, Chapter 2.

59. Felix, R. H. *Mental Illness: Progress and Prospects.* New York: Columbia University Press, 1967, p. 66.

60. *Public Papers of the President of the United States, John F. Kennedy, Containing the Public Messges, Speeches, and Statements of the President, January 1 to November 22, 1963.* Washington, DC: USGPO, 1964, p. 127.

61. Duhl, L. J. The psychiatric evolution. In *Concepts of Community Psychiatry: A Framework for Training*, S. E. Goldston (Ed.). Bethesda, MD: NIMH, Public Health Service Publication No. 1319, 1965, p. 21.

62. Caplan, G. Community psychiatry—introduction and overview. See citation 61, pp. 8–9.

63. Ibid.

64. Lowinger, P. The doctor as political activist, *American Journal of Psychotherapy,* 22:616–623, 1968.

65. Talbott, J. A. Radical psychiatry: An examination of the issues, *American Journal of Psychiatry,* 131:121–127, 1974.

66. Arsenian, J. Toward prevention of mental illness in the United States, *Community Mental Health Journal,* 1:320–325, 1964.

67. Zusman, J. Sociology and mental illness, *Archives of General Psychiatry,* 15:635–648, 1966.

68. See citation 35.

69. Whitaker, L. Social reform and the CMHC: The model cities experiment, *American Journal of Public Health,* 60:2003–2010, 1970.

70. Tischler, G. L. The effects of consumer control on the delivery of service, *American Journal of Orthopsychiatry,* 54:501–505, 1971.

71. Dunham, H. W. Community psychiatry, the newest therapeutic bandwagon, *Archives of General Psychiatry*, 12:303–313, 1965.
72. Ibid., p. 311.
73. Ibid.
74. Ibid., p. 312.
75. Zusman, J. Community psychiatry in 1970: Some successes and failures, *Psychiatric Quarterly,* 44:687–705, 1970.
76. Bachrach, L. L. A conceptual approach to deinstitutionalization, *Hospital & Community Psychiatry,* 23:573–578, 1978.
77. Mosher, L. Research on the psychosocial treatment of schizophrenia: A summary report, *American Journal of Psychiatry*, 136:623–631, 1979.
78. Talbott, J. A. Toward a public policy on the chronic mental patient, *American Journal of Orthopsychiatry*, 50:43–53, 1980.
79. Cypress, B. K. Office visits to psychiatrists: National ambulatory medical care survey: U.S. 1975–1976, *Advance Data from Vital and Health Statistics of the National Center for Health Statistics.* Washington, DC: DHEW Public Health Service No. 28, August 25, 1978, p. 3.
80. Regier, D. A. *The Psychiatric Center Director: An Endangered Species.* DHEW (ADAMHA) Memorandum #42. Washington, DC: DHEW, June 23, 1978.
81. Ibid.
82. Borus, J. F. Issues critical to the survival of community mental health, *American Journal of Psychiatry*, 135:1029–1035, 1978.
83. Bellak, L. Community mental health—ten years later. In *A Concise Handbook of Community Mental Health,* L. Bellak (Ed.). New York: Grune and Stratton, 1974, p. 2.
84. See citation 77.
85. Wynne, L. C. Current concepts about schizophrenics and family relationships, *Journal of Nervous and Mental Diseases*, 169:82–89, 1981.
86. Stein, L. I., and M. A. Test. Alternatives to mental hospital treatment. I. Conceptual model, treatment program, and clinical evaluation, *Archives of General Psychiatry*, 37:392–397, 1980.
87. See citation 75.
88. Goldston, S. E. Selected definitions. In *Concepts of Community Psychiatry,* S. E. Goldston (Ed.). Washington, DC: DHEW, 1965, pp. 195–203.

89. Mustard, H. *An Introduction to Public Health.* New York: Macmillan Co., 1944.

90. See citation 42, Chapter 2.

91. Kennedy, J. F. *Message from the President of the United States Relative to Mental Illness and Mental Retardation, House of Representatives Document No. 58, 88th Congress, 1st Session, February 5, 1963.* Washington, DC: USGPO, 1963.

92. See citation 26, Chapter 2.

93. See citation 89.

94. Feldman in citation 89.

95. Feldman, R. H. Foreword. In Caplan, G. *Principles of Preventive Psychiatry.* New York: Basic Books, Inc., 1964.

96. See citation 95.

97. Felix in HEW Task Force on the Report to the President from the President's Commission on Mental Health: *DHEW Publication No. (ADM) 79-848.* Washington, DC: DHEW, 1979.

98. Caplan in citation 97.

99. Zusman, J. Primary prevention. Secondary prevention. Tertiary prevention. In *Comprehensive Textbook of Psychiatry, Vol. II.* A. M. Freedman, H. I. Kaplan, and B. J. Sadock (Eds.). Baltimore: Williams and Wilkins, 1975, pp. 2326–2345.

100. Davis, J. A. *Education for Positive Mental Health: A Review of Existing Research and Recommendations for Future Studies.* Chicago: Aldine Publishing Co., 1965.

101. See citation 97.

102. *Task Panel Reports Submitted to the President's Commission on Mental Health. Appendix Report of the Task Panel on Prevention. Vol. IV.* Washington, DC: USGPO, 1978, pp. 1822–1963.

103. See citation 97, p. G-5.

4

REAPPRAISAL AND RECOMMENDATIONS

In this final section we shall summarize the development of the CMHC program—its conceptual flaws, problems with implementation, and the recent effects of reduced funding. Then we shall review the successes of the Community Mental Health movement and of the CMHC program that, along with the disappointments, have made distinctive contributions to the theory and practice of modern psychiatry. We shall conclude with suggestions for mental health care and for the directions that community psychiatry might take if it heeds the lessons learned.

SUMMARY OF CMHC PROGRAM

During this century there has been a trend away from the hospital toward community care of the mentally ill. By 1955, when more than 558,000 persons were in State or County mental hospitals,[1] public willingness to accept greater responsibility for the mentally ill was marked by the establishment of the Joint Commission on Mental Health and Illness and later by the CMHC legislation of the early 1960s.

The CMHC program of the 1960s—a new service pattern for the care of the mentally-ill—was created in response to a need and was promoted by the climate of public opinion. It was based on the successes achieved by early community psychiatry programs, many of which were in operation in the 1950s. Spear-

61

headed by leaders in community psychiatry, most of those early community programs had evolved in response to local problems and had been put into action creatively and carefully. The CMHC program of the 1960s, however, was launched with much enthusiasm but without sufficient testing and without either the requirements or the means for scientific evaluation.

Conceptual Flaws

The hastily designed CMHC program was handicapped from the start by conceptual flaws stemming from unrealistic views of the community and of mental health. Those related to the concept of the community were:

- The belief that traditional, sharing communities still existed throughout the nation and were the fundamental units of societal organization;
- The notion that catchment areas, defined solely by the numerical size of the population, were "communities"; and
- The overrating of the ability of these "communities" to: (1) care for or "absorb" the severely mentally ill, (2) administer and eventually fund the CMHCs, and (3) control their own destinies insofar as mental health was concerned.

The concept of mental health in vogue during the 1960s produced semantic confusion and other difficulties. The emphasis on mental health rather than on mental illness resulted in a priority for primary prevention at the expense of care for the mentally ill. It also fostered the belief that minimally trained people and indigenous personnel could deal with problems in the community more effectively than professionals.

In Chapter 3, we discussed nine major assumptions fundamental to the CMHC program. All of them are appealing, but there is little scientific evidence of the validity of most of them.

Excessive Expectations

Expectations of the new CMHC program were too high. Optimism about mental health led to an underestimation of the complexity and chronicity of most mental illnesses and to a lack of awareness of the burden that mental illness places on the family and on the community.

Other unrealistic expectations were:

- The idealization of the "right" to receive care;
- The conviction that CMHCs should, and could, do everything for everybody, even establish secure living conditions; and
- The hope that mental illness would cease to be a formidable problem because primary prevention would reduce its incidence and science would find cures for the remainder.

Problems

The CMHC program soon ran into difficulties. It showed the strain of having two masters: on the one hand, the distant Federal Government's overregulation and bureaucratic rigidity, and on the other, inexperienced local citizen boards which often were subjected to pressures from various political groups in the community. Other problems with implementation at the local level were produced by disruptive quarrels among the staff about status and territoriality.

During the 1970s, the CMHC program continued to expand without evaluation or the flexibility needed to meet changing needs, to tailor services to the realities of diverse localities and centers, or to correct apparent failures. Only about one-half of the envisioned 1,500 centers were established. By the late 1970s, many of the existing CMHCs were in financial difficulty aggravated by the progressive phasing out of Federal grant support. In addition, the economy, both nationally and in many states, was ravaged by inflation and by growing unemployment. In many parts of the nation, the taxpayers voted against increasing taxation. The election of 1980 showed that a conservative trend was sweeping the country. As financial support dwindled, many CMHCs were forced to reduce programs and services and in some instances to shut down entirely.

In the meantime, over-reaching into the community and over-expansion of programs had attracted new populations to mental health services. The entire service system was quickly overloaded with the "worried well" who sought treatment while deinstitutionalization was rapidly increasing the numbers of seriously and chronically ill patients in the community. At the same time, other special unserved or underserved patient groups such as children, the elderly, and the chronically mentally ill did not receive needed attention.

In the 1980s, the CMHC program was modified by the Mental Health Systems Act that "reaffirmed" a commitment to the concept of community care and to the states as service coordinators and program raters.[2] The new Act abandoned one of the central features of the original CMHC legislation—that individual communities should shape their programs with direct Federal funding. It was hoped that coordinated funding at the State level would "avoid a system in which the community, the State, and the Federal levels operate in isolation or in two-level collusion."[3] The new Act marked the end of the first phase of the CMHC program in which a new mental health service delivery system was established.

Uncertainty about the future of the CMHCs has been increasing. The Mental Health Systems Act was not funded in 1981. There were justifiable fears not only that the block grants from the Federal Government to the states would reduce the overall funding level for CMHCs, but also that the CMHCs might not receive their share of the already limited financial support. Some CMHCs intensified their efforts to attract paying patients and curtailed services to the indigent. At present, the CMHC program is in a critical condition and may not survive if funding is diminished even more. Many politicians supported the CMHC program when it was expedient to do so but abandoned it when "social programs" became unpopular.

Thus, the already beleaguered CMHC program has had to cope with the problems produced by drastically reduced funding. During periods of conservatism, social programs, particularly those aimed at improving the quality of life for the disadvantaged, are limited, if not eliminated. Of such programs, those for the care of the mentally ill are usually the first to be sacrificed; the stigma of mental illness persists and, as a group, the mentally ill are not a forceful political constituency. In conservative eras, the climate of opinion tends to rely more on social control mechanisms to contain the mentally ill than on programs for their treatment and care. The medical historian, Henry Sigerist, has shown that the role of the sick, the role of the physician, and the practice of medicine are primarily aspects "of the general civilization of the time and are largely determined by the cultural conditions of that time."[4]

Successes

In our reappraisal of Community Psychiatry we have focused on the problems that have dogged the Community Mental Health movement and the CMHC program. Our seemingly harsh assessment has been motivated by the wish to uncover reasons for the disappointment in order to avoid a repetition of past mistakes as we plan for the future.

We emphasize, however, that some of the CMHCs have worked well, especially those located in communities with populations and resources that fitted the Community Mental Health movement's leaders' preconceived views of the community and their models for mental health care. Others that have worked well are centers that have grown "organically," developed slowly but progressively in accord with the needs of the community and the availability of resources. A number of these have never sought or obtained Federal funding. Although they may have started with Federal categorical requirements in mind and with hopes for Federal funding, they have had to rely primarily on their own resources. An excellent example is provided by the rural outreach programs fanning out from the Texas State hospitals.[5] They are not Federally supported; instead, they compete with Federal CMHCs for state dollars. Many of these facilities and others like them have been more responsive to local needs than the Federally-funded and regulated CMHCs because they have retained flexibility. Consequently, they have constructed community linkages and have concentrated on what is needed locally rather than on Federal guidelines. Some of these small local programs express great pride in their independence.

Ingredients of Success. First of all, we now know that effective community care is feasible for many patients who, fifty years ago, would have been consigned to a life of oblivion in the back wards of dreary mental hospitals. From studies of successful individual community care programs and the experiences of those that have been disappointing, we can identify some of the ingredients making for this success:

- consistent and adequate funding
- assignment of top priority to the needs of the most seriously ill
- accessibility of services
- availability of a full range of treatment and rehabilitation measures for individual patient needs
- responsiveness to expressed local needs as opposed to categorical needs
- effective interagency communication and planning
- maximum use of existing community resources and the development of new resources for demonstrated service gaps
- active involvement of psychiatrists as caregivers and planners

- use of well-trained professionals for providing both services and supervision
- internal harmony among the staff
- pursuit of staff development and "anti-burnout" strategies
- encouragement of active participation of the private psychiatric sector in patient care
- objective assessments of needs and well-designed program evaluations.

Contributions to Mental Health Care

Beyond its immediate consequences for the care of individual patients, the Community Mental Health movement has had important effects on the traditional organization of mental health care. The old-fashioned State hospital has become far less isolated. Not only has it opened its doors to the families of the mentally ill and to interested citizen groups, but it has changed its organizational structure to include a variety of services—partial hospitalization, after-care, out-reach programs—within its own facilities and in the community it serves. All of these advances and services, especially when they are coordinated and where there is continuity among the various caretaking units, provide improved therapeutic approaches to patients. And further, these advances make local care accessible to those who need it. As a consequence of the extension of services into the community, the citizenry, having become more familiar with the nature of mental illness, is somewhat more tolerant and understanding of the afflicted.

* * * * * * * *

In retrospect, we can view the CMHC program as an experiment in mental health care that has had constructive as well as disappointing outcomes. How well it has worked is a question about which we can only speculate. The number of patients in residence in State and County hospitals, 558,992, was at its height in 1955, almost ten years before the CMHC program was established. In 1978, there were approximately 147,000 hospitalized patients. But, the prophecy that many of these patients would neither be treated more effectively nor "cured" by relocation in the community has been at least partially confirmed by the tremendous increase in readmissions—the "revolving door." The number of admissions has almost tripled in three decades, from 152,286 in 1950 to about 414,000 in 1980. The greatest decrease in the number of patients in residence and the greatest increase in admissions both occurred in the 1960s. If the transfer of patients from the hospital to the community had not been so precipitous, is it possible that better resources and techniques for reducing admissions—often readmissions—might have evolved? The most serious and persisting problem, attributable to the decline of the State hospitals and to the lack of funding of social programs, is that a large number of the chronically mentally ill are often lodged in inadequate nursing homes and board-and-care facilities in the community or, even worse, in single uncared-for rooms, and are not receiving needed treatment. An increasing number of the mentally ill are in jails or prisons and, in our larger cities, many of them wander aimlessly through the streets.

The rate of the movement from institutional to community care appears to be slowing both in the United States and the United Kingdom. Recently, the Royal College of Psychiatrists stated:

> It is only since 1957 that the concept of care of the mentally disordered within the community became accepted policy.... The subsequent development has been uneven and decisions have been taken, based more upon intuition than knowledge, research, and experience.[6]

The phenomenal growth of the outpatient practice of psychiatry during the last two decades has been accompanied by the steadily increasing development of psychiatric units in general hospitals in the community. Although, unfortunately, there are still many mentally ill who go undiagnosed and receive no treatment, large numbers of them are being cared for in the offices of private practitioners, in non-Federally-funded community facilities, or episodically in general hospital emergency rooms.

In its early days, many prominent psychiatrists were eloquent voices for the CMHC program; but as its problems multiplied, enthusiasm waned and community psychiatrists did not supply sorely needed leadership. The result has been demedicalization and a progressive withdrawal of psychiatrists. In recent years, psychiatrists have more often been critics than advocates of the CMHCs. At present, most CMHCs are headed by non-psychiatric administrators and are staffed mainly by social workers and other mental health professionals, a large number of whom have had limited training. Generally, the few psychiatrists are primarily engaged in prescribing medications and carrying out medical functions so that CMHCs can qualify for Medicaid and other Federal funding.

Although community psychiatry has not developed as a subspecialty, many psychiatrists are working in the community in appropriate traditional and innovative settings. The principles and practices of community psychiatry have been incorporated into the general practice of psychiatry. In this respect, there is a parallel between the development of community psychiatry and of consultation-liaison psychiatry. Neither has become a subspecialty but the "compleat" psychiatrist has had training in community psychiatry and in consultation-liaison work; it is now taken for granted that he or she can work effectively in the community as well as in the general hospital or a private office.

Finally, we must recognize the vital influence that the Community Mental Health movement and the CMHC program have had on the training and professional activities of all psychiatrists. Psychiatric residents are now exposed to a broad spectrum of learning experiences—24-hour emergency rooms, crisis intervention, partial hospitalization, family diagnosis and therapy, community consultation and education—that provide them with a wide armamentarium of therapeutic techniques they can subsequently carry with them into practice. Perhaps most important of all, psychiatrists have learned that the assessment of the patient's functional capacity is as important a determinant of therapeutic management as the symptom diagnosis; the concept of rehabilitation has become an equal partner with that of acute treatment. The CMHC program has called attention to the importance of sociocultural factors in the definition, course, and treatment of mental illness—an emphasis that is especially needed at present when many psychiatrists are fascinated by the successes of biological psychiatry. Psychiatrists, indeed, have expanded their awareness to include a recognition that illness, in Engel's terms, is truly a biopsychosocial phenomenon.[7]

As we reappraise community psychiatry and look toward its future, we can see that although psychiatrists and others had unrealistic expectations of the CMHC program twenty years ago, the program overall has benefited community psychiatry. The extension of psychiatric care into the community was a needed countervailing force to the predominance, on the one hand, of psychoanalysis and long-term office treatment and, on the other, of custodial care that often led to the social breakdown syndrome and chronicity.

RECOMMENDATIONS

Community psychiatry, the Community Mental Health movement, and the CMHC program have had a major impact on modern American psychiatry. Even the disheartening and disillusioning effects of the past quarter of a century take on importance when we view them as cautionary tales. We conclude, therefore, with several recommendations derived from our reappraisal for the organization of future mental health programs.

Geographic service areas must take political realities, natural boundaries, and transportation networks into account. These criteria are more important than mere numbers of people. Since, as we have learned, "communities" rarely exist as such, programs should seek to identify natural constituencies and their leaders to gain assistance and support.

Future programs need to be designed—flexibly, not rigidly— to meet the needs of the community, with due regard for the availability of resources. The goals of community mental health can be pursued in a variety of settings, not just in Federally-funded CMHCs. The increasingly evident limitations of resources require us to select from a wide variety of potential programs those that are considered to be most essential and that can be established with reasonable assurance of continued support. Future efforts ought to emphasize the treatment and rehabilitation of the mentally ill rather than reliance on preventive strategies or broad social programs of unproved effectiveness. Our limited resources must be directed primarily toward the alleviation of suffering that results from mental illnesses and their consequences. In this respect, we need to recognize that case finding efforts should be used sparingly, since they tend to increase rather than reduce service demands.

Ongoing evaluations of programs and of therapeutic outcomes should be undertaken in order to correct methods, improve services, and monitor directions. Major investments in service programs should not be made until research has shown what is needed, how goals are to be attained, and whether available resources can be applied effectively. Psychiatrists ought to be involved in the planning, implementation, and monitoring of all programs to prevent the blurring of programmatic focus and the lines of professional responsibility. Finally, the lessons learned from the successes and the failures of the CMHC program should become an integral part of the education of future psychiatrists.

In *summary*, community psychiatry has been a long-standing

part of the field of psychiatry. During the 1950s and 1960s interest in, and optimism about its possibilities burgeoned and possibly outran its potential. The CMHC program, a new and expanded service program, was handicapped from the start by conceptual flaws and by untested assumptions about the superiority of community to hospital care. Moreover, the CMHC program was never fully implemented. It appears that the rigid CMHC program diverted community psychiatry from its developing course; nevertheless, benefits did accrue to the theory and practice of psychiatry and to a better understanding and treatment of the mental illness.

POSTSCRIPT

At this time, it is impossible to foresee the effects of the changes in Federal policies of the early 1980s on the care of mental patients. It would be foolhardy for us to predict the direction such policies will take in the years ahead. Despite these troubling uncertainties, the knowledge gained from our recent experiences with the Community Mental Health movement and the CMHC program is applicable to future programs that may be developed to help the mentally ill in the United States.

REFERENCES

1. NIMH Division of Biometry (personal communication, 1978).
2. See citation 67, Chapter 2.
3. Ibid.
4. *Henry E. Sigerist on the History of Medicine.* F. Marti-Ibanez (Ed.). New York: The Publications, Inc., 1960, p. 24.

5. Texas Department of Mental Health and Mental Retardation. *Basic Standards and Guidelines for Outreach Programs.* Austin: TDMHMR, 1976.
6. *The Mental Health Service After Unification.* Report of the Tripartite Committee of the Royal College of Psychiatrists, the Society of Medical Officers of Health, and the British Medical Association. London: British Medical Association, 1972.
7. Engel, G. L. The need for a new medical model: A challenge for biomedicine, *Science,* 196(4286):129–136, 1977.

ACKNOWLEDGMENTS TO CONTRIBUTORS

The program of the Group for the Advancement of Psychiatry, a nonprofit, tax exempt organization, is made possible largely through the voluntary contributions and efforts of its members. For their financial assistance during the past fiscal year in helping it to fulfill its aims, GAP is grateful to the following:

Abbott Laboratories
American Charitable Foundation
Dr. and Mrs. Jeffrey Aron
Dr. and Mrs. Richard Aron
Virginia & Nathan Bederman Foundation
CIBA Pharmaceutical Company
Maurice Falk Medical Fund
GEIGY Pharmaceuticals
Ethel L. Ginsburg Estate
Mrs. Carol Gold
The Gralnick Foundation
The Grove Foundation
The Holzheimer Fund
The Island Foundation
Ittleson Foundation, Inc., for Blanche F. Ittleson Consultation Program
Marion E. Kenworthy-Sarah H. Swift Foundation, Inc.
Lederle Laboratories
NcNeil Laboratories
Merck, Sharp & Dohme Laboratories—Postgraduate Program
Merrell-National Laboratories
Phillips Foundation
Sandoz Pharmaceuticals
The Murray L. Silberstein Fund (Mrs. Allan H. Kalmus)
The SmithKline Beckman Corp.
Mr. and Mrs. Herman Spertus
E.R. Squibb & Sons, Inc.
Jerome Stone Family Foundation
Tappanz Foundation
van Ameringen Foundation
Wyeth Laboratories